KT-568-618

The National Childbirth Trust
offers information and support in pregnancy, childbirth and early
parenthood, and aims to enable every parent to make informed choices.
Donations to support our work are welcome.

THE PERINEUM IN CHILDBIRTH

A SURVEY OF WOMEN'S EXPERIENCES
AND MIDWIVES' PRACTICES

Wendy Greenshields SRN SCM
Hannah Hulme SRN RM

Edited by Sandy Oliver PhD

Authors and editor worked together as members of the
Research and Information Group of the National Childbirth Trust.
Valuable support and advice was received from other members of the Group.

ISBN 1 870129 49 0

Questionnaire Design
Wendy Greenshields SRN SCM
Diane Mcginlay RGN RM
Jo Moran-Ellis MSc RGN
Deirdre Mackay MSCP (ACPOG)
Heda Borton MSCP (ACPOG)
Mary Newburn BSc
The Royal College of Midwives

Library Service
Patricia Donnithorne HND Pgdip. Lib.
Joy Foottit

Computer Support
Andrew Greenshields Eng. Tech. F.I. Diag.E
Tim Snape (Abbotsbury Software)

Statistician
Helen Billington PhD

Illustrator
Kirsty Greenshields BA

The National Childbirth Trust aims to enable every parent to make informed choices. We are concerned that important aspects of maternity care have not always been thoroughly evaluated and therefore choice is often based on incomplete or inaccurate information.

The NCT recommends that all new procedures and treatments are introduced as research studies which are subjected to rigorous evaluation before being adopted more widely. Current forms of care which have not been adequately investigated for their benefits, risks and side-effects should, where possible, be subjected to equally stringent evaluation and open debate.

Whilst parents may be guided by research evidence, individuals making decisions will be influenced by their own beliefs, wishes and priorities.

©The National Childbirth Trust 1993. All rights reserved. No part of this publication may be reproduced in any form by any means, without the prior permission of the National Childbirth Trust.

Registered No. 2370573 (England)
Registered office: Alexandra House, Oldham Terrace, London W3 6NH
Registered Charity No. 801395

CONTENTS

LIST OF FIGURES

CHAPTER ONE
INTRODUCTION

Aims of the Study

Methods and Limitations

Perineal Trauma: the Extent of the Problem

A Wider Perspective

"I was totally unprepared for the degree of pain which resulted, and the time for which it lasted. All preparation before birth seems to concentrate on labour and the immediate aftermath in terms of emotional/hormonal imbalance. I was not expecting to feel such physical debilitation for a period, counted in WEEKS after the birth. The pain itself was quite serious, but it also caused me mental distress in that I could not care for my baby as I wished to..." - one mother's description of the aftermath of her episiotomy.

This survey is the fourth in a series undertaken by the **Research and Information Group of the National Childbirth Trust (NCT).** Each survey deals with a different aspect of maternity care or parenthood and each is related to concerns expressed by our membership. *The Perineum* in Childbirth* survey was suggested following comments made by members during previous research projects (8,22,46), comments which emphasised the distress caused to many women by a painful perineum following childbirth.

Aims of our Study
The study sought the views of both mothers and midwives. Our aims were:

- To assess the incidence of different types of perineal trauma.
- To determine which factors might influence the type of trauma women experience.
- To discover what measures are taken to promote healing and relieve pain.
- To explore the long term effects of perineal trauma.
- To compare current practice with published research and, if a discrepancy appears, to attempt to discover why research findings are not always applied.
- To identify areas related to perineal care worthy of clinical research of the type that the NCT cannot itself do, but midwives could.

*Glossary of medical and midwifery terms at the end of this booklet.

1

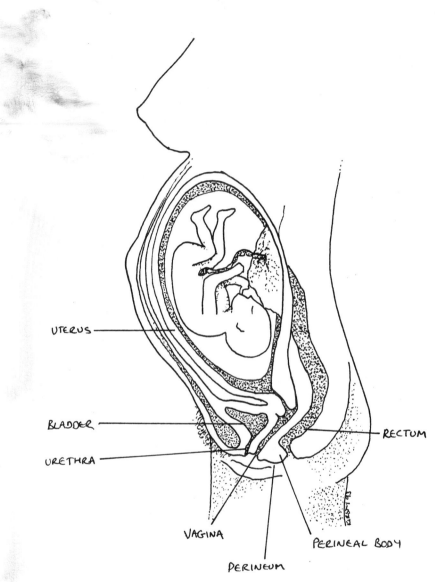

UTERUS

BLADDER

URETHRA

RECTUM

VAGINA

PERINEAL BODY

PERINEUM

Illustration 1: Female internal reproductive organs — cross section.

The perineum is the area between the entrance to the vagina and the anus. It forms the base of the perineal body, which is a wedge-shaped block of tissue made up of muscle, fat and connective tissue and measuring about 4x4x4 cm. The perineal body is flattened by the baby's head (or bottom) as it descends the vagina. At the point of "crowning" the perineal body is therefore thin and easily torn or cut. Immediately after delivery it returns to its usual pyramid-like shape so repair of the area is relatively complex.

Methods and Limitations

We collected information from two questionnaires; the first, for mothers, was distributed through our quarterly journal *New Generation* (45), and the second, for midwives, was printed in *The Midwives' Chronicle* (47), a monthly professional publication. The questionnaires are contained in Appendices 1 and 2 of this survey.

The mothers were asked for details of births which took place in 1990 and the midwives were asked for details of deliveries that they had attended during the month prior to completing the questionnaire. Mothers and midwives were also asked for their views on a range of topics relating to the perineum.

Questions addressed to both the mothers and the midwives focussed on research-based practices which have been reported in midwifery and obstetric journals.

A total of 2334 mothers returned questionnaires. A number were not included in the analysis because the births they related to fell outside the study period of 1990, delivery was by Caesarean section or the questionnaires were returned too late for inclusion in the study. Two thousand questionnaires were analysed. Most of the women, 1672 (84%), were members of the NCT.

A total of 380 midwives returned the questionnaire. Their responses related to their attendance at 2149 births.

Probabilities, calculated using Chi-square statistical tests, are included on all figures where it was possible to calculate such values. Where these tests are significant they have identified a difference in distribution of the incidence of perineal trauma between the groups.

Both samples were entirely self-selected and may not reflect the views and experiences of all women giving birth and all midwives practising at that time. This means that although the results reported here are statistically significant within the confines of our survey, *we do not claim that they necessarily apply to the general population.*

Most of the mothers who responded were NCT members. NCT members are often assumed to be older and better informed than most childbearing women, although we have no evidence to support this assumption.

It may be possible that women who had a particularly difficult experience were more motivated to respond to the survey, although other women may have responded to share the enthusiasm felt following a good birth experience. This said, previous survey experience indicates that women simply like filling in our questionnaires no matter what the topic. Many mothers use the opportunity to "de-brief" their birth, often sharing traumatic experiences for the first time.

A number of the midwives who completed the questionnaire expressed a particular interest in the care of the perineum and pleasure that we were asking the views of midwives. (One or two others wrote to tell us that they would not complete the questionnaire for fear of what "the NCT would do with the information".)

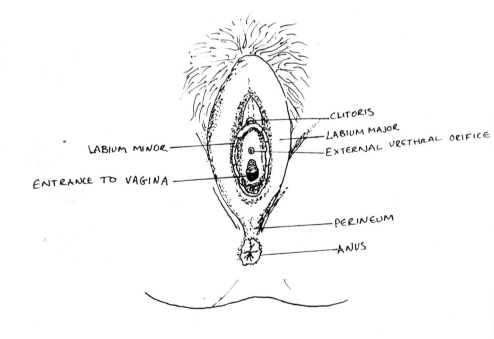

Illustration 2: Female external genetalia.

4

Perineal Trauma: Extent of the Problem

Of the 2000 women included in the analysis of our survey 410 (20.5%) had an intact perineum. Nearly half of the sample, 900 (45%), sustained tears of varying degrees. A further 690 women (34.5%) had an episiotomy, including some who had a tear in addition to an episiotomy. These figures are illustrated in **Figure 1.**

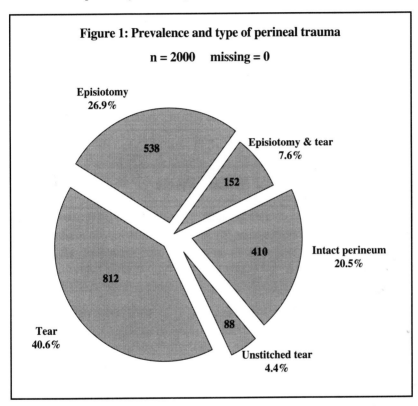

Figure 1: Prevalence and type of perineal trauma

n = 2000   missing = 0

Episiotomy 26.9% — 538
Episiotomy & tear 7.6% — 152
Intact perineum 20.5% — 410
Tear 40.6% — 812
Unstitched tear 4.4% — 88

In addition to the trauma shown in **Figure 1,** 309 women (15%) reported injuries other than to the perineum. Of these tears:

- **53% were of the labia;**
- **20% were vaginal;**
- **9% were of the clitoris;**
- **5% involved the urethra;**
- **3% (10 women) had third degree tears (tears involving the anal sphincter).**

The remaining mothers suffered various combinations of the above, including a tear reaching the anus, a torn cervix, an episiotomy which extended out to the buttock and a perineum described by a GP as "generally shattered".

5

The midwives' reports of perineal trauma experienced by women whom they had recently assisted were markedly different. We averaged out the individual results and noted:

- **an intact perineum rate of 48%;**
- **a tear rate of 39%;**
- **an episiotomy rate of 13%.**
- **In addition, of the women attended by these midwives, 7% experienced tears of the labia, clitoris or urethra.**

Women who had delivered babies before (1026 of the 2000 respondents) experienced less perineal damage than those giving birth for the first time. The effect of pre-birth factors on perineal trauma is discussed in Chapter Two.

Although 80% of women had a normal delivery, our sample included all vaginal deliveries, normal as well as instrumental. Sixteen percent of mothers had forceps deliveries and 4% had a vacuum extraction. Perineal trauma rates for different types of vaginal delivery, and other factors relating to labour, are discussed in Chapter Three.

According to women, the main explanations offered by midwives for *tears* sustained at delivery were:

- **the baby was not in the optimum position for delivery;**
- **the birth happened "too quickly";**
- **the baby was "too big" or the "mother too small".**

Again according to women, the principal reasons given for *episiotomies* were:

- **a forceps delivery;**
- **fetal distress;**
- **to "speed up delivery";**
- **to "avoid a tear".**

We deal further with the explanations given for perineal trauma and the initial repair of injury in Chapter Four.

Chapter Five describes the subsequent care of damaged perinea, whilst Chapter Six looks at some of the long terms effects of this trauma. Chapter Seven comprises a summary of our findings and suggestions for further research.

We outline our recommendations on the prevention and treatment of perineal trauma in Chapter Eight; although these recommendations take note of the experiences of respondents, they are based principally on our review of established research on the subject. Throughout this report, at the end of each chapter, we place our findings in the *Wider Perspective* of other research projects dealing with the perineum in childbirth.

A Wider Perspective

After 1967, when midwives were given approval to perform episiotomies, the episiotomy rate increased dramatically and doubled between 1967 and 1978, rising from 25% to 53%. By 1978 70% of the women having their first baby had an episiotomy (34). In 1981 the NCT published Kitzinger and Walter's Some Womens' Experiences of Episiotomy (31), *which triggered a surge of interest in the subject. Our own survey* Rupture of the Membranes in Labour (8), *published in 1989 but relating to births which took place in 1987, reported an episiotomy rate of 38% and an intact perineum rate of 19%, these figures were based on a self-selected NCT sample, similar to that of this present study and inclusive of all vaginal deliveries.*

Despite our method of sampling, perineal trauma reported in NCT surveys is similar to that described in other UK studies. A literature review (44) reports a very wide variation in rates of perineal trauma. Episiotomy rates in 17 North West Thames Region hospitals in 1990 ranged from 23% to 41% with intact perineum rates of 21% to 41%.

While it is heartening to see a continuing decrease in the episiotomy rate between 1987 and 1990, it is important to note that, according to our own surveys (this one and Rupture of the Membranes in Labour, *mentioned above), the intact perineum rate remains fairly static at around 20%; episiotomies are apparently being replaced by tears. Similarly, restricting the use of episiotomy in a randomised controlled trial also resulted in increased spontaneous trauma, although there was a simultaneous increase in the intact perineum rate from 24% to 34% (53). On the other hand, an audit of midwifery practice from 1981 to 1986 at Northwick Park Hospital showed a drop in the overall episiotomy rate from 39% to 17% accompanied by an increase of equal proportion in intact perinea while tears remained relatively unchanged (32).*

Although the women responding to our questionnaire experienced a relatively high rate of perineal trauma, we were encouraged by the figures presented by the midwife respondents. These figures refer only to normal deliveries but, even so, it is good to see what can be achieved by apparently skilled and motivated practitioners. Warren and Kargar (61) propose that midwives take their lead from colleagues such as these who achieve low perineal trauma rates, other midwives could examine these practices in order to improve their own.

CHAPTER TWO
BEFORE THE BIRTH: FEARS AND FEELINGS

The NCT Sample: Age and Previous Babies

Feelings during Pregnancy: Views on Episiotomies and Tears

Sharing these Views with Midwives

Preparation during Pregnancy: Perineal Massage

A Wider Perspective

" The perineum was described by the physiotherapist 'was not quite the worst she had ever seen'.... How I ever dared to conceive a second - it did take me four years to pluck up the courage and my excessive silliness during pregnancy my GP attributed partly to fear of a repeat birthing." - a mother writing about her feelings during her second pregnancy.

The NCT Sample: Age and Previous Babies

The mothers ranged in age from 17 to 43 years, the mean age being 29, median 30 years. We could discern no link between maternal age and perineal injury.

In spite of the tendency for subsequent babies to be bigger we found that the more babies a mother had delivered, the less likely she was to have an episiotomy and the more likely she was to have had an intact perineum **(Figure 2).**

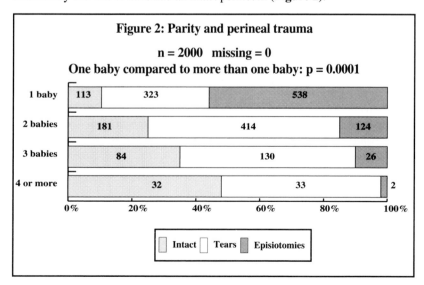

Figure 2: Parity and perineal trauma

n = 2000   missing = 0

One baby compared to more than one baby: p = 0.0001

8

Feelings during Pregnancy: Views on Episiotomies and Tears

We asked the women if they had had opinions on episiotomies and tears *before* their babies were born. 1410 mothers gave us their views and these are illustrated in **Figure 3.**

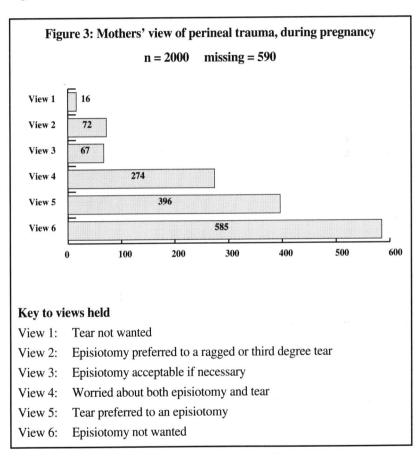

Figure 3: Mothers' view of perineal trauma, during pregnancy

n = 2000   missing = 590

View 1	16
View 2	72
View 3	67
View 4	274
View 5	396
View 6	585

Key to views held

View 1:   Tear not wanted

View 2:   Episiotomy preferred to a ragged or third degree tear

View 3:   Episiotomy acceptable if necessary

View 4:   Worried about both episiotomy and tear

View 5:   Tear preferred to an episiotomy

View 6:   Episiotomy not wanted

The following are typical quotes:

"Having had an episiotomy with the first, was desperate not to have another."

"I was terrified of tearing (wanted an episiotomy with local)."

"Wanted to avoid episiotomy if at all possible."

"Would have preferred an intact perineum."

9

When we compared the views expressed by women with the trauma they *actually experienced*, an interesting pattern emerged as shown in **Figure 4.**

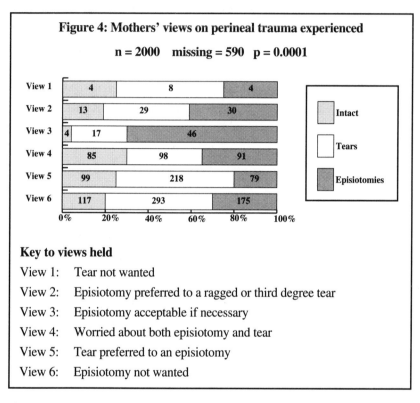

Figure 4: Mothers' views on perineal trauma experienced

n = 2000   missing = 590   p = 0.0001

Key to views held

View 1:   Tear not wanted

View 2:   Episiotomy preferred to a ragged or third degree tear

View 3:   Episiotomy acceptable if necessary

View 4:   Worried about both episiotomy and tear

View 5:   Tear preferred to an episiotomy

View 6:   Episiotomy not wanted

Those women who appeared *least concerned* about episiotomy prior to the birth had by far the *highest* episiotomy rate, about half of them having the procedure performed. Likewise, those who said they preferred a tear to an episiotomy actually had the highest tear rate, whilst women who were worried about tears *and* episiotomies had the highest intact perineum rate.

Given the evidence, it seems likely that the midwives involved may have been mindful of the mothers' wishes; women were more likely to have an intact perineum if that was what they wished. Or is it possible that women who most consciously want to avoid perineal trauma behave differently during labour and so directly influence the degree of trauma they experience? We also noted that women who were not particularly opinionated on the subject of perineal trauma were more likely to have an episiotomy. Perhaps in the absence of an expressed wish from the mother, some midwives prefer to do an episiotomy.

Alternatively, these figures may be a product of a retrospective survey, women having tailored the views they thought they held prior to the birth to fit in with what actually happened. These responses may therefore be part of the process of coming to terms with this part of their birth experience. A prospective study would clarify the influence of women's views before birth on their subsequent experience.

Sharing these Views with Midwives

We asked women if they had been able to discuss their views with their midwives prior to delivery and then compared their responses with the perineal trauma they experienced **(Figure 5).**

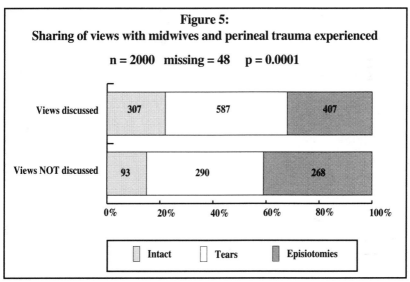

Figure 5:
Sharing of views with midwives and perineal trauma experienced

n = 2000   missing = 48   p = 0.0001

We found that women who wished to avoid perineal trauma were more likely to achieve this if they were able to discuss their views with their midwives before the birth; clearly midwives were responsive to the wishes of mothers. Once aware of a mother's wishes, the vast majority of midwives preferred *not* to perform episiotomies; many went to great lengths to work with mothers to achieve an intact perineum. These quotes are representative of many we read:

> *"The doctor and midwife encouraged me to try almost anything I think to avoid an episiotomy."*

> *"My midwife....knew exactly what I wanted from our chats beforehand and she was excellent."*

It may also be that women who are assertive enough to raise the question with their midwives are also more likely to follow their own wishes and instincts in labour, which may result in a better perineal outcome.

11

Sadly, we were also told of situations where communication between midwives and labouring women was either impossible or ignored:

> "....the new midwife arrived as Sarah's head was emerging - hence I didn't get a chance to discuss anything until she was delivered. I do feel that if I had been attended by the same midwife for all of the second stage I would have had less problems with tearing."

> "I had had an injection before the birth because the midwife said she would have to give me an episiotomy. I objected strongly but she replied that it would be necessary - no reason given."

A number of women said that they *could* have discussed their views if they had wanted to, but chose not to do so for various reasons. These reasons included having written a birth plan, knowing the midwives from a previous delivery or simply trusting their attendants' professional judgement.

Preparation during Pregnancy: Perineal Massage

Perineal massage is described in a paper published in the *Journal of Nurse-Midwifery* (5):

> "Massaging the perineum...daily for the last 6 weeks of pregnancy may help avoid the need for an episiotomy and/or prevent tearing by reducing resistance in the vaginal and perineal tissues...The massage should be done daily for 5-10 minutes beginning 6 weeks before you are due....You can do the massage yourself, using your thumbs, but it is probably easier for your partner to do this with you....Massage a natural oil...into the tissues of the perineum and lower vaginal wall.....As you massage each night, your tissues should relax and stretch...."

Just over a fifth (22%) of women practised perineal massage during pregnancy in an effort to minimise trauma during childbirth. At first sight this technique appeared to make very little difference to the outcome, but when we considered just first time mothers having normal deliveries the effect became more apparent, as **Figure 6** indicates. However, because practising perineal massage was a personal choice for each woman we cannot identify a causal relationship between perineal massage and an intact perineum; for this a randomised controlled trial would be necessary.

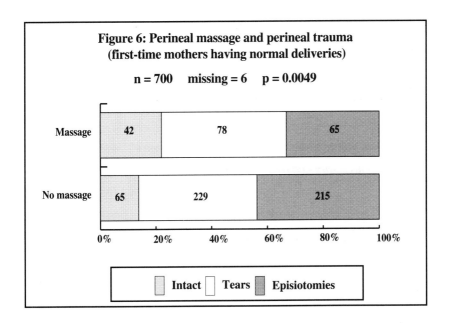

Figure 6: Perineal massage and perineal trauma
(first-time mothers having normal deliveries)

n = 700   missing = 6   p = 0.0049

We asked the midwives their views on perineal massage during pregnancy. Nearly a fifth of the midwives (19%) felt that antenatal massage helped preserve the perineum. Some (18%) said they taught mothers how to massage their perinea during pregnancy, and a few more (20%) thought the *mothers* felt it was worth doing.

A Wider Perspective

Our survey showed a gradual increase in intact perinea and a gradual decrease in episiotomies with increasing parity. In their randomised controlled trial of 1000 women, Sleep et al (53) likewise found a higher incidence of intact perinea and a decreased incidence of episiotomies in multiparous women compared with primiparous women.

In this survey antenatal perineal massage was associated with higher rates of intact perinea only when it was practised by women expecting their first baby. Previous studies have also reported an association between perineal massage and a reduction in episiotomy rates (4,5,14) but Avery and Van Arsdale (5) concluded that more research is needed. Despite a lack of conclusive evidence that perineal massage helps to preserve the perineum, articles have already appeared in popular "mother and baby" magazines describing the technique (3,7).

Of the women in our survey, 59% would be prepared to practise perineal massage in future pregnancies; 33% might do so and 7% would not. This said, we still do not have any indication of the number of women who would be prepared to be randomised in a clinical trial designed to test the effects of perineal massage.

CHAPTER THREE
THE BIRTH AND THE BABY

".....the single most important contributory factor was the presence of a midwife that I liked/respected/felt that she cared. The first time I felt like a caged animal. This time I felt in safe hands and even though I tore, it healed quickly - she sewed it so carefully and the whole experience was wonderful. No depression afterwards - I could sit down! No ice packs. I feel much less of everything would be needed if one could have midwives who cared and made the mother feel safe and loved." - a mother describing her second delivery.

Place of Birth

We asked women where they delivered their babies; at home, in a general practitioner (GP) unit, a hospital consultant unit, or elsewhere. The majority (78%) of the 2000 mothers gave birth in a consultant unit. Of the remaining women, 206 (10%) birthed at home and a further 185 (9%) used a GP unit. The degree of perineal trauma experienced varied widely between different places of birth. Women who delivered at home were the most likely to have an intact perineum and the least likely to have an episiotomy - as indicated in **Figure 7.**

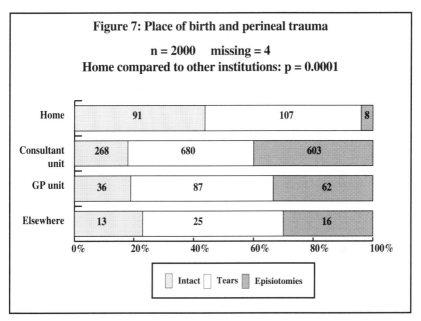

Figure 7: Place of birth and perineal trauma

n = 2000   missing = 4

Home compared to other institutions: p = 0.0001

We initially questioned whether these differences might be attributed to the increased incidence of operative deliveries in hospitals and to the smaller proportion of women giving birth to their first baby at home. We therefore compared just first time mothers having normal deliveries with their place of birth (**Figure 8**). Although the number of women having their first baby at home was quite small, their experience appeared to confirm the original observation that a greater proportion of women giving birth at home keep their perinea intact. However, we do appreciate that this difference may be due to a combination of factors, such as relative freedom from medical protocols, differing midwifery practice and differing wishes and behaviour of the labouring women.

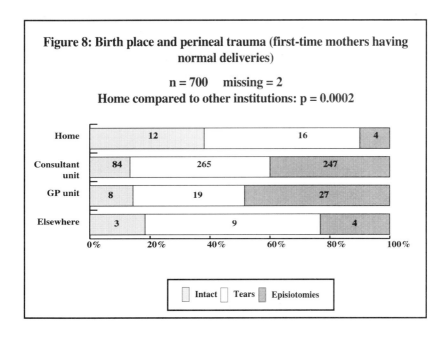

Figure 8: Birth place and perineal trauma (first-time mothers having normal deliveries)

n = 700   missing = 2
Home compared to other institutions: p = 0.0002

Birth Attendants

- 88% of the deliveries were attended by midwives;
- 1% by GPs;
- 7% by hospital doctors;
- 4% by "others". The "others" included midwifery and medical students, ambulancemen, husbands - and even the odd policeman! Ten women did not tell us who attended them during their deliveries.

Of the 410 women who had intact perinea, 92% were delivered by midwives. Of the 135 women delivered by hospital doctors, 93% were given episiotomies. These figures are consistent with policies which allow midwives to attend normal deliveries while doctors attend forceps deliveries and vacuum extractions.

We did, however, explore the difference that individual *midwives* can make by asking them in their questionnaire about their use of episiotomy in a normal labour. Their replies are illustrated in **Figure 9.**

16

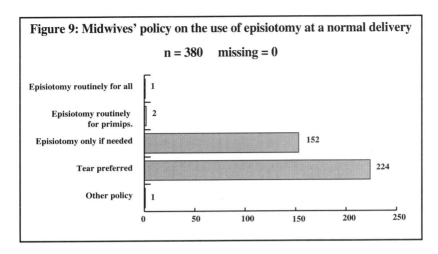

Figure 9: Midwives' policy on the use of episiotomy at a normal delivery

n = 380   missing = 0

As these figures demonstrate, over half of the midwives felt that a tear was generally preferable to an episiotomy, and, as **Figure 3** indicates, most women fear episiotomy above other perineal trauma. We explore the after-effects of both tears and episiotomies in Chapters Five and Six, but would like to acknowledge at this point that for some women an episiotomy is not necessarily a negative outcome, as these two mothers describe:

> *"I had an episiotomy on the birth of my first child having pushed for two hours. It was a relief when it was performed and I had started to tear apparently. The episiotomy healed quickly and neatly....with my second child...I tore. The scar from the tear appears more extensive than the episiotomy, and took a lot longer to heal. It has also not healed neatly."*

> *"I was pleased to have an episiotomy during each delivery, despite the bad press they give to episiotomies generally. Both my daughters had fairly large heads (37 cms circumference) at birth and I had great difficulty in getting them out. Their father said the perineum looked 'shiny and fit to burst' prior to delivery. The episiotomy caused the immediate emergence of the head. I must say that each episiotomy was stitched with no further problem and minimal discomfort."*

First Stage of Labour: Duration and Freedom of Movement

The length of the first stage of labour seemed to have little bearing on perineal trauma, unlike the length of the second stage (see Figure 13). However, the degree of freedom of movement allowed *throughout* labour appeared to make a difference to the trauma experienced as **Figure 10** shows.

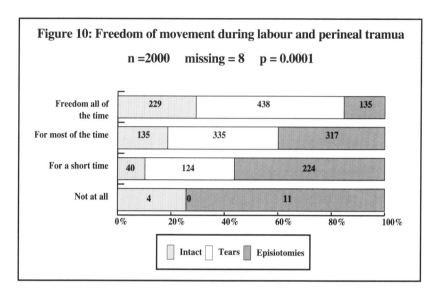

Figure 10: Freedom of movement during labour and perineal tramua

n =2000   missing = 8   p = 0.0001

Freedom all of the time	229	438	135
For most of the time	135	335	317
For a short time	40	124	224
Not at all	4	0	11

☐ Intact   ☐ Tears   ▨ Episiotomies

Two-fifths of the women had freedom to move throughout their labours, while another two-fifths were free to move "most of the time". Women with intact perinea and unstitched tears were far *more* likely to have had freedom of movement for the whole of their labours compared to mothers with tears requiring sutures. Conversely, mothers who had episiotomies were far *less* likely to have had freedom of movement throughout their labours. Speaking generally, we were pleased to note that the majority of women (80%) had freedom of movement at least "most of the time" during their labours.

Epidurals, Operative Deliveries and Rupture of Membranes

Mothers who had epidural anaesthesia were very much more likely to have an episiotomy than those who did not.

Of the 305 women who had an epidural:

- **58% had an episiotomy;**
- **12% had an episiotomy with a tear;**
- **22% incurred tears;**
- **9% had an intact perineum.**

53% of these mothers had either forceps or Ventouse deliveries; 67% of the episiotomies accompanied an operative delivery.

It is encouraging to note that nearly half (47%) of women having an epidural subsequently had a normal delivery.

On the subject of assisted or operative deliveries in general, we noted that vacuum

18

extraction - or Ventouse delivery - is less widely used than forceps, although quite a number of women reported that Ventouse delivery was unsuccessfully attempted before recourse to forceps. One third of vacuum extractions were accomplished without recourse to an episiotomy, the mothers sustaining tears instead. Even delivery by forceps did not mean an automatic episiotomy; just over a quarter of the women having forceps deliveries had a tear instead, with one woman even keeping her perineum intact. See **Figure 11.**

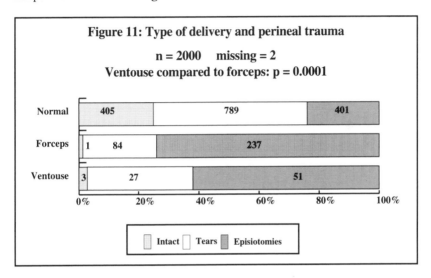

The amniotic membranes of 51% of the women ruptured spontaneously and 42% had their membranes ruptured artificially. A further 7% experienced both spontaneous rupture (probably of the hindwaters) and artificial rupture of the forewaters.

The *type* of membrane rupture was of little significance; it was the *timing* that appeared to tie in with the degree of perineal trauma; rupture during the second stage of labour, whether spontaneous or artificial, was associated with preservation of the perineum compared with rupture during the first stage (**Figure 12**). This association may be a product of midwifery practice and the wishes and behaviour of women, rather than of physiological effect.

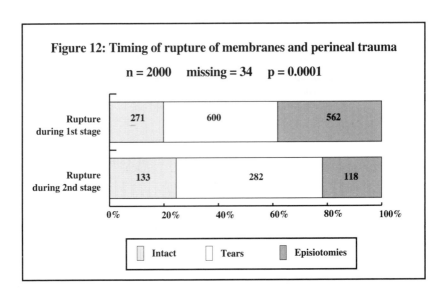

Figure 12: Timing of rupture of membranes and perineal trauma

n = 2000   missing = 34   p = 0.0001

Second Stage of Labour: Duration and Time Limits

We found that when a woman's second stage of labour was longer than 30 minutes she was more likely to have an episiotomy and less likely to have an intact perineum (**Figure 13**).

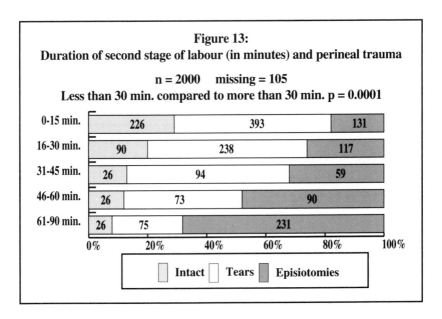

Figure 13:
Duration of second stage of labour (in minutes) and perineal trauma

n = 2000   missing = 105
Less than 30 min. compared to more than 30 min. p = 0.0001

With this in mind we wondered if midwives were still obliged by unit policies to expedite a lengthy second stage, perhaps by recourse to episiotomy. We therefore asked the midwives, first, how long they allowed women having their first baby to push in the second stage and, second, how long they allowed women having second or subsequent babies to push. In *both* instances the vast majority of midwives reported that they were not tied to arbitrary time limits, provided, of course, that all was well with mother and baby (**Figure 14**). However, as we have seen from earlier analyses (see *A Wider Perspective* at the end of Chapter One) the midwives who responded to our questionnaire were not a group representative of those midwives who cared for the women in our survey, as the intact perineal and episiotomy rates of the two samples varied considerably.

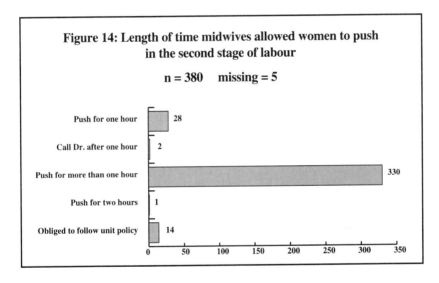

Figure 14: Length of time midwives allowed women to push in the second stage of labour

n = 380   missing = 5

It is possible that the midwives caring for the women in our survey worked under unit policy guidelines to use episiotomy to prevent long second stages. If this is the case, a long second stage alone does not mean that episiotomy becomes more necessary. It would be interesting to look at the length of second stage in homebirths where the intact perineum rate is generally high and episiotomy rate is low, but unfortunately numbers were insufficient in the present survey.

Stand and Deliver?

When we analysed the effect of the delivery position on the perineum we took into consideration episiotomies and *all* tears; labial, vaginal, clitoral and urethral. The results are shown in **Figure 15.**

21

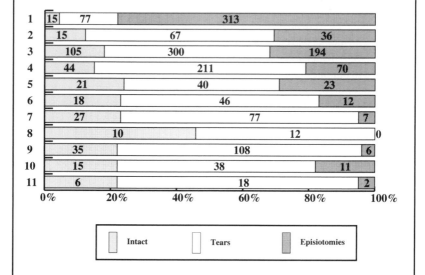

Figure 15: Delivery position and perineal trauma

n = 2000   missing = 21

Standing up (8) compared to on back, propped up (3): p = 0.0004
Standing up (8) compared to kneeling (9): p = 0.030
Standing up (8) compared to supported half squat (10): p = 0.037

Key to positions

1: Flat on back, legs in stirrups or placed on midwives' hips

2: Flat on back, feet on bed

3: On back, propped up

4: Sitting upright

5: On side

6: On side, propped up

7: On all fours

8: Standing up

9: Kneeling

10: Supported half squat

11: Full squat

22

The figures show that the lowest incidence of intact perinea and the highest incidence of episiotomy occurred when a mother was lying flat on her back with her legs either in stirrups or supported on the hips of the two midwives. This may be less of a reflection on the position itself but rather because so many operative deliveries were conducted with mothers in this position.

By far the best outcome was for mothers adopting the standing position; nearly one half (46%) of the 22 women standing had a totally intact perineum, the rest sustained tears and none had an episiotomy. However, it is unlikely that a midwife would attempt an episiotomy while a mother is standing up, and we do not know how many mothers had to abandon a standing position in order to have an episiotomy performed. Unfortunately, only 22 women stood to deliver their babies; a much larger sample would be needed to fully evaluate this birth position.

The position that was associated with the highest level of *tears* was kneeling, with an incidence of 73%; closely followed by the full squat, with 69% of the squatting mothers sustaining tears. Although these positions compare less favourably with standing, when compared with women in the supported half squat, on all fours, on side and on side propped up, the high tear rates in these groups reflects fewer episiotomies, as the intact perineum rates were very similar.

We asked midwives if they had a particular position which they preferred women to adopt for delivery. Just under half of the midwives (139 out of 380) told us their favourite position for delivery and these preferences are shown in **Figure 16.** It is interesting to note that, in spite of their relatively high intact perineum rate (see the end of Chapter One), none of the midwives favoured standing for delivery.

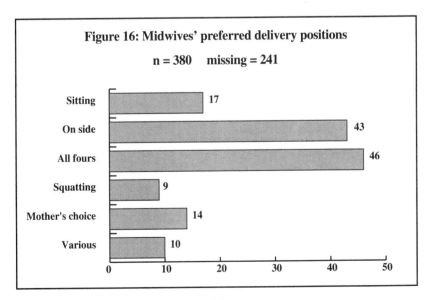

Figure 16: Midwives' preferred delivery positions

n = 380   missing = 241

It may be that if women are allowed freedom to follow their own instincts, to choose their own delivery position and to push as their bodies tell them, that this increases the chance of an intact perineum. Unfortunately, we did not ask the women in our survey specifically about their freedom to choose their delivery position so it was not possible to analyse this idea. Again it is interesting to note that even amongst the midwives who answered our questionnaire, only 10% preferred to allow the mother her own choice of delivery position.

Delivery Instructions

During the 1960s and '70s, midwives tended to organise the delivery of babies with loud and clear instructions to "push push push" followed, at the appropriate moment, by "pant pant pant", an approach sometimes described as "cheerleading". We were interested to find out if this method still prevailed in the 1990s so we asked the mothers four questions about what instructions they were given by midwives during the second stage of labour. The questions, the replies and the apparent effect on perineal trauma are shown in **Figures 17, 18, 19 and 20.**

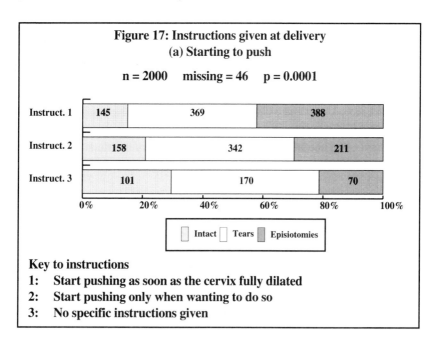

Figure 17: Instructions given at delivery
(a) Starting to push

n = 2000   missing = 46   p = 0.0001

Key to instructions
1:   Start pushing as soon as the cervix fully dilated
2:   Start pushing only when wanting to do so
3:   No specific instructions given

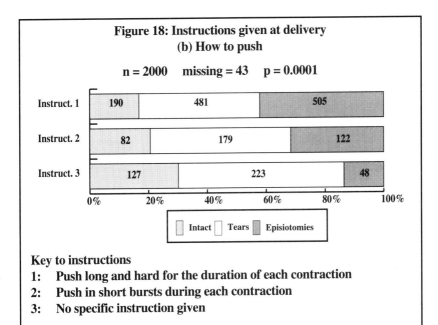

Figure 18: Instructions given at delivery
(b) How to push

n = 2000   missing = 43   p = 0.0001

Instruct. 1   190   481   505
Instruct. 2   82   179   122
Instruct. 3   127   223   48

0%   20%   40%   60%   80%   100%

Intact   Tears   Episiotomies

Key to instructions
1:   Push long and hard for the duration of each contraction
2:   Push in short bursts during each contraction
3:   No specific instruction given

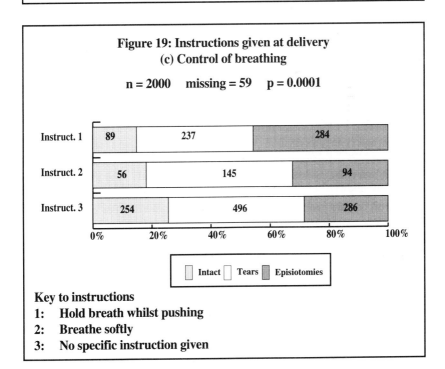

Figure 19: Instructions given at delivery
(c) Control of breathing

n = 2000   missing = 59   p = 0.0001

Instruct. 1   89   237   284
Instruct. 2   56   145   94
Instruct. 3   254   496   286

0%   20%   40%   60%   80%   100%

Intact   Tears   Episiotomies

Key to instructions
1:   Hold breath whilst pushing
2:   Breathe softly
3:   No specific instruction given

25

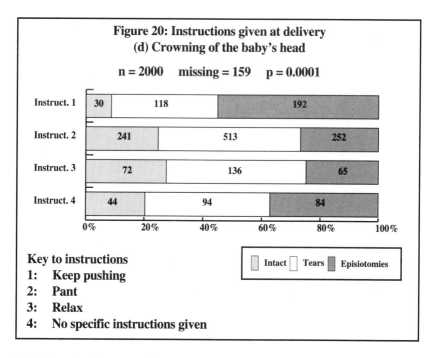

Figure 20: Instructions given at delivery
(d) Crowning of the baby's head

n = 2000   missing = 159   p = 0.0001

Key to instructions
1:    Keep pushing
2:    Pant
3:    Relax
4:    No specific instructions given

In the first three instances (**Figures 17, 18 and 19**) the *less* instruction a mother was given the *better* her chances of having an intact perineum as opposed to an episiotomy. It seems that allowing a mother to "listen" and respond to the sensations of her own body, rather than attempting to impose order on her actions, is more likely to lead to an intact perineum.

The fourth question (**Figure 20**) revealed the one instance where instruction appeared to *increase* the likelihood of an intact perineum and *minimise* the risk of an episiotomy; women who were asked to "relax" or "pant" fared best.

Replies to a corresponding question addressed to the midwives revealed that two-thirds of the midwives encouraged the mother "to push only as she wants to" and only one-fifth encouraged her "to push with every contraction for as long as she can".

Many of the mothers in our survey added descriptions of how they and their birth attendants worked in tandem to minimise perineal trauma:

> "(We tried)...breaking the waters, massaging the perineum, relaxing, pushing, helping me to squat more, change positions etc. until the baby's heart rate dropped for the third time, when we all agreed an episiotomy would be best for all concerned."

"On arriving at the maternity unit we were able to discuss how we would like our labour to proceed with Gill, our midwife. She stated her philosophy - minimum intervention, minimum internals, any delivery position we wanted and no episiotomies except in exceptional circumstances - we were thrilled and felt an instant rapport. While I was pushing Gill massaged my perineum and used her fingers as a focus for me to push against, telling me to push her fingers out. I managed to hold the head on the perineum by panting, gentle breathing and a great deal of encouragement but eventually my son's determination to be born took over and I did tear. Gill was mortified and apologised profusely saying that she had very much wanted to avoid a tear.....Adam's birth was such a joy, the whole experience can truly be described as great fun." (Midwife's name changed).

Significantly, in these two examples, although the mothers experienced trauma they were, in fact, happy with their experiences, since they felt their birth attendants had been sympathetic and had worked hard to try to preserve the perineum.

Delivery of the Baby's Head

We asked midwives if they used manual pressure to help flex the baby's head. This technique encourages the fetal head to tilt forwards so that a relatively narrow diameter of the skull emerges first from the vagina. The results are summarised in **Figure 21.** We did not ask midwives if they also manipulated the vaginal tissues, as recommended by Thompson (57).

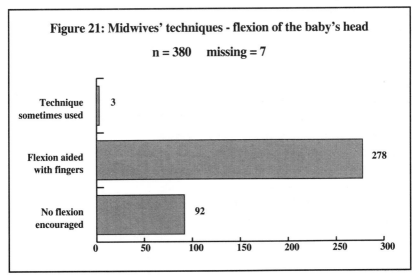

Figure 21: Midwives' techniques - flexion of the baby's head

n = 380   missing = 7

Technique sometimes used	3
Flexion aided with fingers	278
No flexion encouraged	92

One midwife described a slightly different method.

> *"In some cases at the perineal phase, when the head is crowning one can sometimes 'rock' the head through, the only way I can think to describe that, is intermittently flexing in co-operation with the mother and her pushing."*

Thompson (57) also advocates "supporting" the perineum manually during the second stage. We asked midwives about *their* technique (**Figure 22**), but unfortunately we were unable to assess the effect of either of these techniques on the perineum; confirmation, or otherwise, of Thompson's suggestions would require a randomised controlled trial.

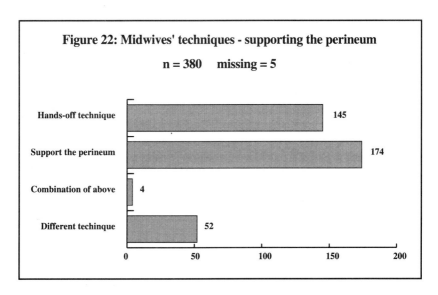

Figure 22: Midwives' techniques - supporting the perineum

n = 380   missing = 5

Perineal Massage

Massaging the perineum during labour appears to be an old midwifery "trick of the trade" which we thought had largely been forgotten. In fact, 150 mothers (7.5%) reported that their midwives used perineal massage in order to stretch the perineum, although statistical tests revealed no significant association with an intact perineum.

In our survey of midwives 11% said they massaged the perineum during labour and 10% thought doing so helped to preserve the perineum.

Waterbirth

In this study, around a fifth of the mothers spent some time in a birthing pool or bath during their labour but this made little difference to the type of perineal trauma experienced.

Only 29 women actually *delivered* while still in the water, so it is difficult to analyse the effect that this type of delivery may have on the perineum.

- **41% had an intact perineum;**
- **45% had a stitched tear;**
- **10% had an episiotomy;**
- **3.5% an episiotomy and tear.**

While these figures look promising the findings are not statistically significant.

The Baby: Gestation and Birthweight

The completed gestations of the mothers in our sample ranged from 26 weeks to 45 weeks, with most, 746, delivering their babies after 41 weeks of pregnancy. The preterm births, i.e. prior to 35 weeks of pregnancy, had high rates of episiotomy; otherwise no discernible pattern of perineal trauma emerged. An episiotomy is often performed for a preterm birth to protect the baby's fragile skull.

Surprisingly, the weight of the baby at birth also appeared to make very little difference. The exceptions were mothers of babies who weighed under 6lbs (2.7kg); their episiotomy rate was 44%, compared with 25% for mothers of babies in the 7-8lbs (3.2kg-3.6kg) range and 33% for the mothers of 8-9lb (3.6kg-4.0kg) babies. The first figure is almost certainly due to the larger number of premature babies in the lowest weight range.

A Wider Perspective

In summary, our survey found that an intact perineum was associated with labours which included features such as:

- **intact membranes during the first stage of labour;**
- **freedom of movement;**
- **minimum of instruction during the second stage;**
- **spontaneous delivery (i.e. without forceps or Ventouse);**
- **giving birth standing up;**
- **giving birth at home.**

Factors which are recognised features of many high technology deliveries, such as epidural anaesthesia, forceps, Ventouse and lying flat to deliver babies, were associated with episiotomies.

Our finding, that minimal instruction during the second stage is associated with preserving the perineum, supports the work of Kitzinger and Simkin (30). In their book "Episiotomy and the second stage of labour" they conclude that "spontaneous (short and intermittent) maternal bearing down efforts alternated with breathing, stretch perineal tissues more gradually than prolonged breath holding and straining, and also allow for better fetal oxygenation". Reported elsewhere, a randomised trial (42) has compared women pushing spontaneously with women instructed to "take a deep breath, hold it and push for as long and hard as possible." Many women in this trial did not push according to the instructions to which they were randomly allocated. As the analysis of perineal trauma was according to the pushing method used rather than the pushing method as allocated, this study cannot guide midwives as to how they should advise women they attend. A search of randomised controlled trials (44) found only one other very small study published of pushing methods in the second stage. Therefore we would like to see a trial randomising women to groups who are either given no instructions during the second stage of labour except to "pant" or "relax" at crowning of the baby's head, or given the usual encouragement to push.

Bearing in mind our own finding that adopting a squat (or kneeling) for delivery seemed to be associated with less chance of an intact perineum compared with standing, it is interesting to read the comments of Dunn (15): "When both thighs are flexed, as they are in the full squat, the introitus is pulled forward and the perineal muscles put in tension. This is fine for defaecation with the small diameter of the stool, but definitely unfavourable for childbirth, as it means the baby must go further round the corner and downward gravity pushes the head against the now tense perineum causing pain, some resistance to childbirth and making perineal tears much more likely."

A recent literature review of randomised controlled trials relating to care of the perineum at delivery concluded that there is no particular benefit, or hazard, resulting from the upright or the recumbent position in relation to the perineal outcome, although there is a decreased risk of episiotomy when upright (44).

Our observation that mothers who had second stages lasting longer than 30 minutes were more likely to have episiotomies is consistent with the possibility that some longer second stages are speeded up by the use of an episiotomy. However, Sleep, Roberts and Chalmers, after reviewing the available evidence, say: "There is no evidence to suggest that, when the second stage of labour is progressing and the condition of both mother and fetus is satisfactory, the imposition of any arbitrary upper limit on its duration is justified. Such limits should be discarded" (54). Caldeyro-Barcia agrees: "Another advantage to a longer second stage is that it gives the perineum more time to stretch slowly and the need for episiotomy is markedly reduced" (11).

One midwifery technique aimed directly at preservation of the perineum is flexion of the baby's head as it emerges. This is advocated by Thompson (57). Thompson's method also involved careful manipulation of the vaginal tissues while the head is crowning. He found that using this technique increased the intact perineum rate from 15% to 69%, while reducing the episiotomy rate from 78% to 7%, although these findings were not within the context of a randomised controlled trial.

There is little published research on the effect on the perineum of delivery under water. Our own numbers are too small to be of statistical value, although it is interesting to note that Burns and Greenish (10) found, in their audit of practice of deliveries in water, a considerable reduction in episiotomies with very little difference in intact perinea and an increase in second degree tears.

Finally, on the subject of assisted deliveries: in a randomised controlled trial of 264 women, Pusey et al reported that significantly more women having a forceps delivery suffered "unbearable perineal pain" at three or four days postnatally compared with women having vacuum extractions (43). These findings, along with those of others (60) lead us to expect a change in the proportion of women having forceps deliveries and vacuum extractions in the future.

CHAPTER FOUR
MAKING GOOD? - REPAIRING THE DAMAGE

When and Who?: Waiting Times and Practitioners

How?: Use of Local Anaesthetic and Suturing Techniques

With What?: Suturing Materials

Why?: Explanations Given for Episiotomies and Tears

A Wider Perspective

"I wish I had been more prepared for the pain AFTER the delivery, stitching up and the fact that part of me would never return to "normal" - or be the same as before - perhaps I was rather naive." - a mother's reply to part of our questionnaire.

When and Who?: Waiting Times and Practitioners

Women reported that perineal damage was generally repaired very quickly; nearly three quarters of the mothers (73%) were attended to within the first half hour after birth. Of those that waited longer, a number said that it had been their own choice to spend some time with their babies before they were sutured. Here is one mothers' comment:

"I sustained a second degree tear to my perineum. I didn't feel the tear as my baby was born with one push...I was sutured within five minutes as a doctor was present at the delivery - quite by chance. I feel the quick suturing contributed to the fast healing and relatively pain free postnatal period."

We asked the women who repaired their tears and episiotomies. Their replies are shown in **Figure 23.**

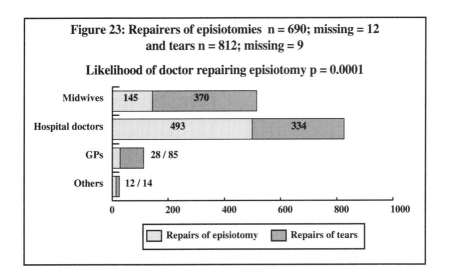

Figure 23: Repairers of episiotomies n = 690; missing = 12
and tears n = 812; missing = 9

Likelihood of doctor repairing episiotomy p = 0.0001

Of the midwives who responded to our questionnaire 66% repaired tears and 60% repaired episiotomies. However, only 45% of the women in our survey who experienced tears and just 21% of those with episiotomies had their perineum repaired by a midwife - relatively small proportions even assuming that doctors perform perineal repairs following operative deliveries. On the other hand, perhaps we should not be surprised at this apparent inconsistency, since, as noted in the Introduction, our sample of midwives was self-selected, many professing a special interest in the subject. Even so, we were disturbed and puzzled that although midwives are now being encouraged by local policies to undertake perineal repair, so few of the profession actually seemed to do so.

Suturing the perineum has, for many years, been an integral part of a midwife's professional training and role. The *Midwives' Rules (58)* and *Code of Conduct (59)* have at no time stipulated that a qualified midwife should not suture; it is simply that the practice has until now been actively or passively discouraged by the policies of most maternity units. Learning how to repair the perineum actually became a requirement of midwifery training in January 1983 when the European Community Midwives Directives came into force.

Reasons for not suturing were given by 142 of the midwives:

- **just under 80% said that it was either because they had not received appropriate post-basic training or were not yet considered competent to suture unsupervised;**
- **10% said that "unit policy" did not allow them to suture;**
- **one midwife said she was allowed to suture and was competent, but that it was more usual for the doctor to perform this task.**

One midwife commented without explanation:

"Perineal discomfort is a major problem in the postnatal period and partly due to the fact that the majority of midwives are not suturing."

Does this midwife feel that midwives would be more skilled at suturing than other practitioners? Or is her belief simply further evidence in favour of continuity of carer? Certainly if an individual attendant is able to offer maternity care throughout pregnancy, birth and the postnatal period she will be well aware of how perineal pain can affect both mother and baby. In addition, her observations may lead her to identify aspects of her practice which could be investigated further or improved on, with the aim of maximising the comfort of women in her care.

How?: Use of Local Anaesthetic and Suturing Techniques

Virtually all the women who needed sutures were given some form of analgesia prior to suturing unless they already had an effective epidural. A third (37%) were given an injection of local anaesthetic. "Entonox" was frequently used, often in combination with local anaesthetic. The remainder of the women were given general anaesthetic, pudendal block, spinal blocks, local anaesthetic spray or valium.

Although most mothers were given pain relief if they needed it, prior to being sutured, we received a number of disturbing reports:

"Having the episiotomy repaired was absolutely horrendous. I consider that my pain threshold is fairly high but despite pain relief by injection into the perineum area prior to stitching, it was the most painful experience of my life."

"By far the most painful part of an easy, even enjoyable birth, was the stitching. This was done firstly by a midwife - inexperienced in stitching - who did the stitches too tightly. It was extremely painful, even with a local anaesthetic, and then the stitches had to be re-done. A doctor, using a stronger anaesthetic, did the second stitching; this was quick and painless. Surely the midwife should use a stronger anaesthetic too."

"My only complaint was that the midwife did not wait for the local anaesthetic to work before starting sewing."

"The one thing I was not happy about was that I was not given further pain relief before stitching - I did feel it and can still remember the pain - I didn't know at the time that I could have been given a whiff of gas and air and that may have helped."

Some mothers found that the position they were forced to adopt for suturing added to their distress.

"I found it degrading lying on a bed with my legs up in stirrups; extremely painful and long - it took about thirty minutes and was the last thing I wanted to be doing at that time."

When questioned about their use of saline or local anaesthetic to infiltrate the perineum prior to suturing when there is an epidural providing effective anaesthesia, nearly a third of the midwives did not answer the question. The remainder replied as follows:

- **3% infiltrated with normal saline;**
- **19% used a local anaesthetic;**
- **49% said they did not infiltrate with anything in these circumstances.**

Please read the final paragraph of *A Wider Perspective* at the end of this chapter for an explanation of the rationale behind this question.

The method of suturing also varied between midwives, as shown in **Figure 24.**

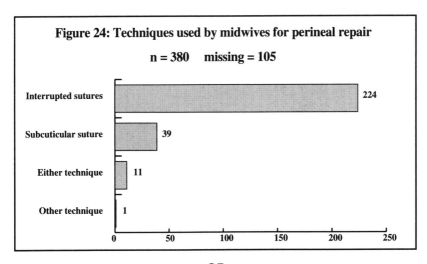

Figure 24: Techniques used by midwives for perineal repair

n = 380   missing = 105

When we asked the midwives why they chose their preferred method of suturing, we were given 37 different answers. A quarter (25%) of midwives said they used the method they had originally been taught; others told us that hospital policy dictated their practice in this area.

Interrupted sutures were preferred by many midwives because they felt that wounds closed this way drained more easily, reduced the risk of a haematoma developing and healed more quickly. Furthermore, they believed that it is harder for infection to spread along an interrupted suture line. The fact that individual interrupted sutures could be removed if they were too tight was also considered an advantage. Other replies contradicted each other, for example, both interrupted and subcuticular sutures were said to be less painful postnatally.

Of the mothers who sustained tears at delivery (45% of those who completed our questionnaire), a tenth reported that their tears were not sutured, presumably because they were relatively small or superficial. We did not explore this topic further in our survey. With hindsight this is perhaps a regrettable omission, since it seems that some midwives are now questioning the need to suture even some second degree tears of the perineum. Professionals holding this view may feel that many tears heal as well, or better, if left free of stitches; could the unique anatomy of the perineum be sufficient to encourage the edges of a wound to come together and rejoin correctly? This was certainly a view expressed by at least one of our respondents:

"After the birth of my son I was told I had a very small tear and that I hardly needed stitching. Eventually I was given approximately six stitches, only one being external. Three months later I was still suffering acute pain on attempting sexual intercourse and some bleeding. Six months later, although the stitches are finally healed I have a lump of scar tissue at the base of the entrance to my vagina which means I have to use local anaesthetic before love-making. Obviously this makes relations between my husband and myself very strained and unspontaneous and I feel that perhaps if I had been allowed to heal naturally without stitches matters might be considerably better."

This hypothesis would, of course, need to be properly evaluated before any recommendations for practice could be made.

With What?: Suturing Materials

At the time of the survey catgut was the most commonly used material for suturing the perineum. 41% of our midwives said that they used it, while 13% said they used Dexon or Vicryl, the trade names for polyglycolic acid sutures. The remainder used a mixture of various silks, nylons or glycerol impregnated catgut.

Over a third (38%) of the midwives stated that their main reason for using a particular suturing material was either that it was "the only one available" or it was "hospital policy to use it". Others claimed that their chosen suture material was the most soluble, the easiest to use or the most comfortable for mothers. Some midwives gave "research-based evidence" as their reason, but did not cite specific papers.

Why?: Explanations Given for Episiotomies and Tears

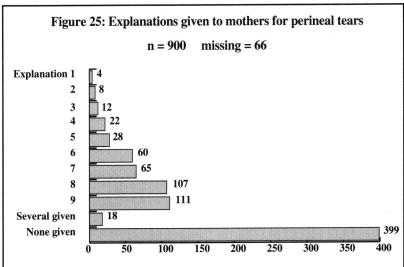

Figure 25: Explanations given to mothers for perineal tears

n = 900   missing = 66

Explanation 1: 4
2: 8
3: 12
4: 22
5: 28
6: 60
7: 65
8: 107
9: 111
Several given: 18
None given: 399

Key to explanations
1:   Delivery by forceps or Ventouse
2:   Tear due to mother's position or actions/inactions at delivery - including one woman who wrote "Used a birthing chair ... bound to lead to being ripped. *It was my fault*" (our emphasis)
3:   Tear allowed in preference to episiotomy
4:   "Poor control in second stage" - not specified whether on part of midwife or mother
5:   Perineum "unyielding"
6:   Old scar gave way
7:   Baby "too large" or "mother too small"
8:   Rapid or sudden delivery
9:   Baby not in a good position at delivery

37

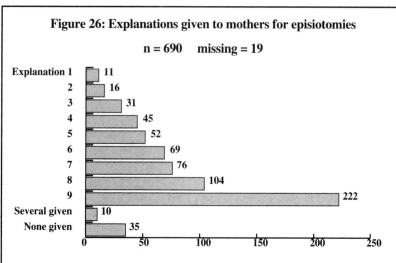

Figure 26: Explanations given to mothers for episiotomies

n = 690   missing = 19

Key to explanations

1: Maternal condition or request (This includes three women who were apparently told that they were "not pushing hard enough" or "pushed at the wrong moment")
2: Scar from previous episiotomy unyielding
3: Baby premature or not in a good position at delivery
4: Baby "too large" or "mother too small"
5: Perineum "unyielding"
6: Episiotomy done to avoid a tear
7: To speed up or facilitate delivery
8: Baby "in distress"
9: Delivery assisted by forceps or Ventouse

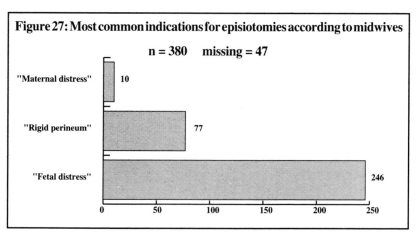

Figure 27: Most common indications for episiotomies according to midwives

n = 380   missing = 47

A Wider Perspective

Important research has been carried out into suturing techniques and materials. Grant (18), in a review of four randomised trials, concluded that women who had their perineum repaired by continuous subcuticular sutures experienced less pain, required less analgesia in the immediate post-partum period and experienced fewer short-term problems than when interrupted transcutaneous sutures were used. Despite these recommendations over half the survey midwives used interrupted sutures, although we were pleased to note that sixteen of the midwives who were originally taught this method were currently learning a subcuticular technique because the result was considered less painful to women postnatally.

In a review of other clinical trials, Grant (18) concluded that "On the basis of currently available evidence, polyglycolic acid sutures (Dexon or Vicryl) should be chosen for both the deep layers and the skin." However, these materials were used by only a minority of our sample of midwives. Research has shown that glycerol-impregnated chromic catgut, compared with ordinary untreated chromic catgut, was associated with significantly more pain at 10 days postnatally and a significantly higher incidence of painful intercourse three years later (56, 19). We would therefore expect to see in future a decrease in the use of this type of material for perineal suturing.

We were disturbed by our evidence that many midwives had continued to use outdated methods and materials for repairing the perineum. This is not necessarily because they are unaware of the appropriate research, rather it may be that they have not been trained in newer methods, are not allowed to use them even if they have been trained, or, simply that the necessary suturing materials are not available for them to use. These are all factors that can be remedied by midwifery managers.

This said, there were apparently midwives who had the necessary materials and who were allowed to do subcuticular suturing, but still preferred to use other techniques. It seems that this was not always a blind rejection of new ideas, but a considered decision based on experience. It may be that a well repaired perineum using interrupted sutures is preferable to a poor subcuticular repair, although whether this idea would be supported by appropriate research remains to be demonstrated.

Research by Khan and Lilford (29) indicates that it is useful to infiltrate the perineum even when there is an epidural still providing adequate anaesthesia. The rationale for this is that infiltration with local anaesthetic or normal saline causes temporary swelling of the tissues which mimics the swelling that normally occurs in the hours following the birth; when the perineum is sutured, this artificial swelling prevents overtight suturing. However, nearly half the midwives completing our survey did not infiltrate the perineum in such circumstances.

CHAPTER FIVE
AFTER THE BIRTH: REMEDIES AND REALITY

Making a Fuss?

Harsh Reality?

Midwifery Support

Oral Analgesia

Remedies

Recommended?: for Relief of Pain

Recommended?: to Promote Healing

Perineal Wound Infections

Self Treatment: Salt and Slippery Elm

Prevention is Better than Cure

A Wider Perspective

"I do feel that some women do not want to make a fuss and tolerate a lot more pain than we are aware of." - a midwife's comment on postnatal perineal care.

Making a Fuss?

The mothers' questionnaires showed a wide variation in the perception of pain postnatally; some women who had an intact perineum were in pain, while two women with an episiotomy *and* a tear had no discomfort!

In general terms, though, women finishing labour with an intact perineum or a tear (whether or not sutures were required) tended to describe themselves as having "slight discomfort" postnatally. Mothers with episiotomy wounds most often said that they had "definite discomfort" (43%) whilst mothers who had an episiotomy and a tear were likely to report that they suffered "pain" (44%).

Harsh Reality?

On the whole, women who had an intact perineum or a tear said that their perineum felt "as expected" or even "less painful than expected". Women with episiotomies, alone or with tears, tended to say that they had experienced "more pain than expected", in fact, 62% of mothers who had an episiotomy with a tear admitted that reality was worse than anticipated.

The distress felt by many mothers is evident in the comments they added to their questionnaires.

"I had quite a nasty tear - borderline third degree, midline - and I never realised, never even considered it could be as painful and unpleasant as it has been, (and still is). While the memory of the birth itself is fading, the memory of the trauma of the tear and the problems it caused (and causes still) is certainly NOT fading! (sic). I couldn't sit for three weeks - not even on a rubber ring - which made caring for a new baby especially awkward. You don't get told that!"

"I must add that although I felt reasonably prepared for the birth, I was shocked at the amount of pain from the stitches (and I had no infection!) and from the bruising around the coccyx."

"I was totally unprepared for how painful my perineum would feel the days immediately following after the birth. All the books you read simply say "you might feel slightly uncomfortable"! and then go on to say how wrapped up you will be in the baby - the inference being that you'll hardly notice the discomfort!"

Thankfully, other women were able to relate happier experiences:

"After my 1st baby (episiotomy and tear) stitched by a male doctor, I had extreme pain for many weeks and slight discomfort up to my second baby's birth. I believe I was stitched too tightly as I had extensive damage from forceps and a big baby....and I was stitched in a hurry. My second baby was born with more force than I would have liked, I don't know if this made me tear badly again or the size of the baby. I had external and internal tears but was unaware of them and didn't realise I'd torn at all until I was about to be stitched. I felt no pain during tearing. I was stitched by the midwife who delivered my baby - she did a wonderful job and I have not suffered a fraction of what I did after my first baby, though the damage was as extensive. I found that just waiting for the tissue to heal was the only remedy but I wasn't as sore as I expected and healed very quickly."

The immediate after-effects of perineal trauma were not restricted to simply localised pain:

"The episiotomy was extensive, skirting the anus - one of the major problems I experienced after the birth was due to very severe haemorrhoids."

"Initially urinating and opening bowels were difficult, more because of anxiety over whether it would hurt. Once I realised it didn't there was no real problem. Similar anxieties are making the first attempts at intercourse tentative, but I envisage no real problems."

Others felt that their preoccupation with perineal problems interfered with their relationship with their babies:

"The dreadful discomfort I experienced also interfered with establishing breastfeeding - I'm sure this may contribute to why some mothers don't succeed - the pain of trying to sit properly is just too much!"

"For the first three months of my baby's life, when a new mother should be enjoying her new baby and when she herself is under great stress with her new role. I was unable to think past the problems I was having with my body and it was as much as I could do to get through one day at a time."

"I didn't sit down to feed my baby for six weeks - and not comfortably for ten weeks."

Midwifery Support

A total of 693 mothers told us that they either sought or were given advice on how to deal with a sore or infected perineum. Most of them (70%) were advised by their midwife. The remaining 30% were advised by doctors, health visitors, physiotherapists, or turned to books, leaflets or the NCT volunteers. A small minority of women (3%) said that no-one advised them.

We were keen to find out how midwives viewed perineal problems in the postnatal period. Is it possible for them to become inured to the pain so many new mothers experience?

Happily this was not the case. According to our survey of midwives:

- **84% regarded perineal pain as a "major problem" for mothers;**
- **13% thought it "a bit of a nuisance";**
- **1% thought it a "very minor problem".**

(Five midwives thought the severity of the problem "varied", while two did not answer the question.)

One midwife wrote:

> *".....perineal discomfort is something that I have been interested in for a long time. To be exact, since the birth of my first child when I found the attitude of my attending midwife to be very matter of fact - "what did I expect?" - and - "just grin and bear it"! So, with this very painful and personal experience in my mind I have tried to be sympathetic and research-based in my practise."*

We wondered if midwives were sometimes too busy to find time to deal adequately and sympathetically with perineal pain. Of the midwives who answered the question:

- **2% said that it was "always difficult" to find time;**
- **54% said it was "sometimes difficult";**
- **42% said it was "never difficult".**

(Five midwives did not answer the question.)

We found that, in general, the greater the perineal trauma, the more time a new mother spent in hospital. The differences were not marked between women with an intact perineum or with tears, it was mothers who had episiotomies who tended to have the longest hospital stays. Of course, this may not always relate to the episiotomy alone, rather to the reason for the episiotomy; for example, a forceps delivery and the additional maternal and neonatal problems associated with this form of delivery. However, if the relationship between perineal trauma and length of hospital stay is a causal relationship, perineal damage has implications for managers, as well as midwives.

We noted that:

- **by the third postnatal day, an average of 66% of mothers with an intact perineum or a tear had been discharged, accompanied by only 38% of the episiotomy group;**
- **at five days, 89% of the intact/tear group had been discharged, but only 74% of the episiotomy group;**
- **at seven days, 99% of the first group had been discharged, compared with 90% of the episiotomy group.**

Oral Analgesia

We asked women about the use of oral analgesia (paracetamol, aspirin, etc.) whilst they were in hospital. Unfortunately replies to this part of the questionnaire were rather incomplete and confused, but we gathered that:

- **28% of mothers accepted pain relief when it was offered;**
- **9% had to specifically ask for analgesia;**
- **2% had to wait over half an hour for their tablets;**
- **0.4% were *refused* analgesia by midwives.**

Altogether, 470 mothers took some type of oral analgesia. Of these women;

- **410 were given paracetamol;**
- **60 were given other drugs, including aspirin, ibuprofen, codeine and co-proxamol. Approximately 10% of the mothers took a combination of analgesics.**

A smaller group of women (399) turned down all offers of analgesia. It may well be that none of these women were actually in pain but we did wonder how many new mothers were anxious about the effects of analgesic drugs on their breastfed babies. As one midwife told us:

> *"Lack of analgesia is something that worries me, especially those mums who are breastfeeding. It is difficult to persuade them that anti-inflamatory drugs are safe."*

Remedies

Mothers were asked if any treatments were applied to the perineum itself to relieve their pain. Nearly two-thirds of mothers (61%) said they did *not* receive any local treatment, whilst 24% said that such therapy was given (16% did not answer the question).

We then asked the women to specify the remedies or treatments suggested by midwives or physiotherapists. The most commonly used topical remedies are shown in **Figure 27.** We were amazed that 588 women described 37 different remedies! (Even that figure is an underestimation since many women reported using a variety of topical treatments grouped together either as "conventional combinations" (ice packs, witch hazel, salt baths, etc.) or "alternative combinations" (homoeopathic and herbal remedies).)

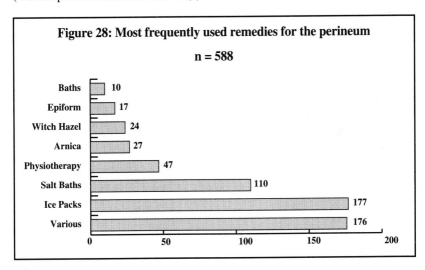

Figure 28: Most frequently used remedies for the perineum

n = 588

The midwives in our survey tended to use an eclectic approach to relieving perineal discomfort and oedema.

The vast majority of midwives (82%) offered a "conventional" range of remedies, including:

- **ice packs;**
- **oral analgesia;**
- **witch hazel;**
- **anaesthetic gels;**
- **Epifoam;**
- **baths;**
- **salt baths.**

Nearly 10% of midwives used an "alternative" approach and their remedies included:

- **calendula;**
- **hypericum;**
- **comfrey;**
- **lavender oil;**
plus some "conventional" remedies.

The remaining midwives reported that they had only a single line of treatment. The most popular was ice packs. Other midwives said they used witch hazel, glycerine packs, different positions to relieve pressure and lignocaine. (The question was unanswered by 13 midwives.)

We asked the midwives in our survey if they were ever required, by senior midwives, medical staff or circumstances, to use treatments which they regarded as outdated or harmful. 12% of midwives agreed that this had happened to them and they listed 25 such remedies, including:

- **salt baths, witch hazel and ice packs;**
- **hydrogen peroxide, Savlon and Eusol;**
- **Epifoam and lignocaine gel;**
- **rubber rings;**
- **Softgut.**

Recommended?: for Relief of Pain

We asked the mothers: "Which remedy or treatment was most effective in *relieving pain*?" and 795 women gave us 68 different answers. These answers can be divided into four groups - thermal treatments, oral analgesics, topical applications and mechanical means of relief.

Thermal Treatments: 24% of women chose some form of *heat* therapy - bath, shower, bidet or other (unspecified) application of warm water. Just under a tenth of mothers (9%) chose *cold* as the best form of pain relief, principally in the form of ice packs although frozen witch hazel pads, ice cold Milton-soaked pads and cold showers were also mentioned.

Oral Analgesia: 18% of women thought that oral analgesia gave the greatest relief from pain; the majority of these women said that paracetamol was the most effective drug on offer.

Topical Applications: 6% of mothers felt that locally applied remedies helped the most. They cited hypericum, calendula, anaesthetic gel and Epifoam. One mother reported using a magnesium sulphate poultice.

Mechanical Relief: 4% of mothers mentioned sitting on rubber rings and cushions.

Various physiotherapy treatments were recommended by a few mothers and "hyperventilating" and "positive thinking" each had their advocates.

Recommended?: to Promote Healing

We asked; "Which remedy or treatment was most effective in *promoting healing?*" This question was answered by 835 women; once again, a wide variety of remedies were favoured:

- **salt baths were recommended by 13%;**
- **regular use of baths, showers and bidets was encouraged by 30%;**
- **"time" was the best healer for 9%;**
- **arnica was favoured by 6%;**
- **various topical treatments including calendula, steroid creams, hypericum, Epifoam and Kamillosan, were advocated by 9%.**

Minority recommendations were:

- **bath additives - various antiseptics, lavender oil, Badedas bath oil and soap flakes;**
- **keeping the wound "clean and dry" (13 mothers);**
- **keeping the wound "moist" (one mother);**
- **using a hairdryer instead of a towel to dry the perineum;**
- **subcuticular sutures;**
- **Dexon sutures;**
- **removal of sutures;**
- **ultrasound;**
- **exercise;**
- **ultimately for one mother, a repair operation.**

Many other remedies were likewise offered; quite a number of mothers suggesting a combination of therapies both to relieve pain and to promote healing.

Perineal Wound Infections

> *"I had an infection which never stopped hurting. I had an infection of my stitches whilst in hospital, the treatment they gave was washing me with antiseptic solution and the removal of one or two external stitches. Ten months later I had a remedial operation and things did improve, although I still couldn't comfortably wear tampons or sit down without being careful until the birth of the second child."* - a mother's description of perineal wound infection.

Perineal wound infections were reported by 157 of the 2000 mothers. **Figure 29** compares the incidence of infection with the type of perineal damage sustained.

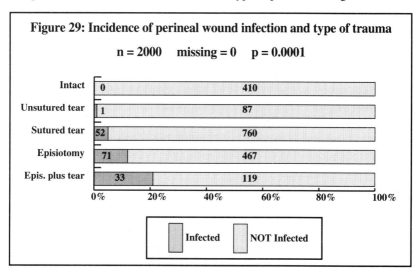

Figure 29: Incidence of perineal wound infection and type of trauma

n = 2000   missing = 0   p = 0.0001

The treatment of infection was described by 136 of the 157 mothers who had infections:

- **43% were prescribed antibiotics;**
- **32% were given a single "conventional" remedy;**
- **13% were given a "conventional" combination of remedies;**
- **11% received "no treatment";**
- **2% were given an "alternative" remedy.**

Most of the midwives in our survey (83%) advised a range of "conventional" treatments when the perineum was infected. These included salt and Savlon baths, Eusol in various strengths, hydrogen peroxide, Providone, Debrisan and a plan to "investigate personal habits and advise accordingly".

An "alternative" range of treatments, including honey, presumably applied locally, was suggested by 5% of the midwives.

Only 6% of midwives said that they saw no infections, or very few in the course of their work.

Throughout this part of the survey we were struck by the sheer diversity of remedies described in both the mothers' and the midwives' questionnaires, although, oddly enough, the range of treatments reported by the women was, in general, quite different to that proposed by the professionals.

Self Treatment: Salt and Slippery Elm

Mothers were asked if they had used any remedies of their own to treat an infected or sore perineum. Of the 2000 mothers, 36% (723) said that they had, and went on to describe 55 different remedies which they had used either singly or in combination.

By far the most popular remedy was arnica (a homoeopathic remedy), used by 19% of the self-treating mothers. Although many mothers did specify that they used arnica tablets, this was not always clear and manufacturers of some formulations warn against the use of arnica ointment on broken skin. Other widely-used self-prescribed remedies were, in descending order of popularity:

- **an "alternative" combination of remedies;**
- **salt baths;**
- **a "conventional" combination of remedies;**
- **calendula ointment;**
- **ice packs;**
- **witch hazel.**

The "alternative" remedies included herbal preparations (hypericum, comfrey, calendula and slippery elm), essential oils (lavender, camomile and tea-tree), staphisagria (a homoeopathic remedy) and "rescue remedy". Other mothers mentioned drinking squaw vine tea, having a bath containing Badedas bath oil, sitting on a semi-frozen sanitary towel or using saliva.

Prevention is Better than Cure

We were interested to find out how much advice new mothers were given on basic perineal hygiene; concerning, for example, keeping the area clean and the correct handling of sanitary towels.

Nearly all of the midwives in our survey (93%) said that they gave such advice to mothers. However, only 53% of the women remember being given any specific advice on perineal hygiene. This discrepancy may merely reflect the fact that the midwives who responded to our survey do not represent the whole of their profession, or possibly midwives really do not give advice as often as they think they do. Alternatively it may be that mothers simply do not recall being advised, or do not perceive what was said to them as advice.

Perhaps as expected, the more damaged a woman's perineum, the more likely she was to be advised on this aspect of her postnatal recovery, 30% of mothers with an intact perineum were advised compared with 64% of those with an episiotomy and tear.

Nearly a half (43.0%) of mothers who were instructed in perineal hygiene received a "range of advice". **Figure 30** indicates the guidance the majority of the women were given.

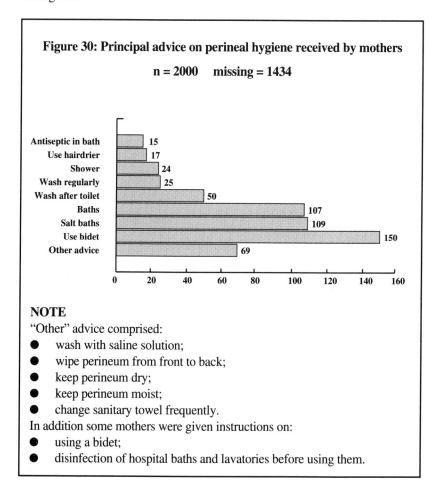

Figure 30: Principal advice on perineal hygiene received by mothers

n = 2000   missing = 1434

NOTE

"Other" advice comprised:

- wash with saline solution;
- wipe perineum from front to back;
- keep perineum dry;
- keep perineum moist;
- change sanitary towel frequently.

In addition some mothers were given instructions on:

- using a bidet;
- disinfection of hospital baths and lavatories before using them.

We were curious to find out if there was any link between perineal wound infection and use or non-use of sterile sanitary towels.

We asked mothers if their hospital provided sanitary towels, and whether these were sterile or non-sterile:

- **22% of women were provided with sterile towels;**
- **5.4% were given non-sterile towels;**
- **51.8% had to provide their own, presumably non-sterile towels.**

(7.4% of mothers did not answer the question).

Respondents reported using sanitary towels from a total of 25 different manufacturers plus supermarket 'own brands'.

The sort of towel used (sterile/non-sterile, hospital-supplied/own) was cross-tabulated with women who had perineal damage, and then with those developing perineal wound infections: there were no significant differences.

It would have been interesting to make further comparisons, for example, between plastic backed and non-plastic backed towels, but this was not possible due to lack of data.

Finally, having waded through such a morass of remedies - from arnica to witch hazel and back again - we were anxious to discover whether there were any possible connections between wound infections and the perineal therapies themselves. The figures in **Figure 31** are drawn from the mothers' questionnaire; they show the substance or hygiene measure used and the number of women using those measures who suffered an infection. These figures are not statistically different, moreover, we do not have information to show whether the remedies were used prior to the onset of infection or in response to infection - so we cannot make any causal inference. We simply offer these figures to provoke thought and, hopefully, provide impetus for randomised controlled trials.

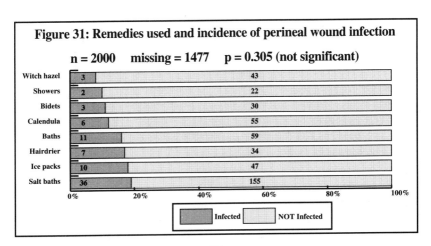

Figure 31: Remedies used and incidence of perineal wound infection

n = 2000   missing = 1477   p = 0.305 (not significant)

A Wider Perspective

Cold Comfort?

In our survey ice packs were the most commonly used topical remedy for relief of pain, although less than 10% of the women thought they were the best form of pain relief. The evidence in research literature on the benefits of ice packs for perineal trauma is confusing because while ice may relieve pain it may also interfere with healing. Rhode and Barger (48), for example, state that "Cold therapy immediately after trauma relieves pain and promotes vasoconstriction to decrease bleeding and oedema, thereby limiting the severity of the trauma. **After 28 to 48 hours, cold therapy may interfere with wound healing"** *(Our emphasis).*

Moore and James (38) proposed that ice does not necessarily provide the best pain relief.

Local Relief

A few mothers mentioned that they had used local anaesthetic sprays or gels to relieve perineal pain. In a review of the evidence, Sleep (50) suggests that lignocaine gel is the most useful as it provides good pain relief at reasonable cost, without the local stinging associated with alcoholic sprays. However, one community midwife told us that in her experience lignocaine gel erodes sutures. No evidence could be found in research literature to support this view, but it may be worthy of further investigation.

Epifoam was used by 17 of the women responding to this survey and was recommended by some of the midwives even though it has been shown to inhibit wound healing and increase the risk of wound breakdown (21).

Rubber, or Sorbo, rings were used by some mothers in our survey, though it has been reported that lymphatic drainage and blood circulation may be adversely affected by the pressure pattern produced (33).

The "Valley Cushion", a pressure-relieving device developed by UT Care Products Ltd., was not in general use at the time of this survey. This cushion is available through the NCT. It offers a "realistic alternative to the ring cushion...(it) has a tapered central channel which allows for adequate perineal circulation and good pressure relief. The supportive sections of the cushion, under each buttock, are separately inflatable and contain special inserts designed to avoid sciatic nerve pressure" (62). The Valley Cushion has been favourably evaluated in a small study in a London maternity unit.

Clean.....?

Some midwives told us that Eusol, alone or with paraffin, was a useful treatment for infected perinea, but others considered this substance to be harmful. Johnson (26) is unreservedly damning: "there is now ample evidence of the dangers of using hypochlorites such as Eusol in open wounds, yet they continue to be used. Hypochlorites have been shown to cause irreversible damage to the micro-circulation, and to interfere with fibroblastic function and collagen synthesis. Furthermore they attack coliform organisms, and release endotoxins. The latter are absorbed, and can produce a range of side effects, varying from mild uraemic toxaemia, to acute renal failure. There are safe alternatives to hypochlorites."

Many mothers in our survey mentioned the importance of plenty of warm baths, but this practice is not necessarily conducive to cleanliness. In "Applied Microbiology" (12) the author states: "when a patient has a bath, he shares it with millions of bacteria from his own skin and gut, to say nothing of those remaining from the previous person. Using a shower exposes a person to lesser risk of cross infection than does using a bath."

Salt baths appeared to be a universal panacea, although Sleep and Grant (52) concluded that there is no case for recommending either salt, or Savlon, in baths. Ayliffe et al (6) could not substantiate claims that salt has either antibacterial or antiseptic properties, but Johnson (28) found one maternity unit using three tonnes each year!

Providone iodine, mentioned by one midwife as a useful topical treatment for perineal wound infections, is described in the British National Formulary (9) as "best avoided" since the iodine can be absorbed by the vaginal mucosa and secreted in breast milk.

Saline rinses and washes were used by some mothers, a practice recommended by Johnson (27). Normal saline has the advantage of being of the same salinity as tissue fluids and should not delay healing or cause irritation.

In a previous survey "Postnatal Infection" (22), the NCT received a number of reports of inadequately cleaned hospitals, conditions which may have contributed to the acquisition of wound infections.

.....and Dry?

Using a hairdryer to dry the perineum seemed to be a common practice. Perhaps the rationale for this is that blowing warm air onto the perineum is a "non-touch" way of drying the area, as opposed to using a towel that might transfer harmful organisms to the wound. However, it is possible that hairdryers may harbour pathogenic organisms, and that infection may actually be transmitted from one woman to another sharing a communal machine. Furthermore, excessive drying of wounds may inhibit healing.

Herbs and Homoeopathy

Herbal and homoeopathic remedies seemed to be very popular amongst the mothers, and midwives, who helped with our survey. Sadly, though, very few of these remedies have been subjected to thorough evaluation.

Witch hazel was included in a randomised trial conducted by Moore and James (38); its value as an analgesic agent was compared with ice and Epifoam. Witch hazel appeared the most effective on the first postnatal day, although ice provided more pain relief on day three, therefore no clear differences were seen overall. Spellacy (55) found that perineal pads soaked in witch hazel and glycerine were no more effective than those soaked in plain tap water.

Gibson et al (16) conducted a double bind trial comparing the effect of arnica (a homoepathic remedy) with placebo tablets when taken by acute trauma patients. Arnica was found to "relieve stiffness and improve general well being" in the vast majority of patients prescribed it but the authors conclude that further larger studies are needed.

Another small study by Hofmeyr et al (24) assessed the effectiveness of two potencies of arnica in relieving post-partum symptoms such as perineal pain and breast pain. The potencies D6 and D30 (equivalent to the x potency in this country) were compared with a placebo; while there was a trend toward D6 being more effective, this study was also too small to be conclusive.

Newer Treatments

Just a few mothers in our survey mentioned the use of ultrasound and pulsed electro-magnetic therapy.

Grant et al (20), in a randomised placebo-controlled trial of both therapies, found that 90% of mothers thought that the treatments had improved their condition. Following ultrasound, perineal bruising looked worse; this then cleared quickly, but with no corresponding relief of pain. Mothers having pulsed electromagnetic therapy reported more pain at 10 days following delivery than mothers having ultrasound therapy. There were no differences in the results of the two treatments three months later. Neither treatment had any effect on perineal oedema or haemorrhoids. In conclusion, the researchers felt that more studies are needed to fully evaluate ultrasound and pulsed electro-magnetic therapy.

Maxwell (35), in a review of research literature, concluded that the effect of therapeutic ultrasound on healing remains unknown and stated that further research is needed to determine the cellular and molecular effects of ultrasonification.

Research

While considerable research has been conducted into antenatal and intrapartum care, relatively little work has been done on the postnatal period. What little has been done does not appear to have significantly affected midwifery care of the traumatised perineum. Harris' study into the practice of 76 individual midwives in a district general hospital concluded that "important research findings were not applied.....the majority of the reported practice was not research-based" (23). Fortunately, the book "Postnatal Care" edited by Alexander, Levy and Roch (1), does much to redress the balance by drawing together pieces of research on which to base care. This book is an excellent resource for midwives, especially when they are advising mothers who are tempted to try some of the multitude of remedies already discredited by research. It may also give support to those midwives who admitted in their questionnaires that they are required to use treatments which are "outdated or harmful".

CHAPTER SIX
BACK TO NORMAL?

Feeling "Normal" Again
"A Miracle I Ever Became Pregnant Again"
Neurotic?
Wise Before the Event?
Stress Incontinence: Who Suffers?
Stress Incontinence and the Birth
Control of Flatus
A Wider Perspective

"Doctors might say "It's early days yet" and women might confess it took a year before they felt back to normal, but its no consolation when your own tear - or part of it- has healed but is still horrifically painful. When is the cut-off point between slow but normal healing and something which has healed but has been incorrectly sewn up?!! I can't believe my vagina is ever going to improve as it is - the perineum tear has improved greatly, however I am seeking medical advice on the sex problem. I feel I need to see a specialist as I'm sure something must be wrong. It's all very well for the doctor to say 'early days', but when sex is so painful that penetration is impossible and brings one to tears with pain, it can't be alright." - taken from a letter one women wrote to accompany her questionnaire.

Feeling "Normal" Again

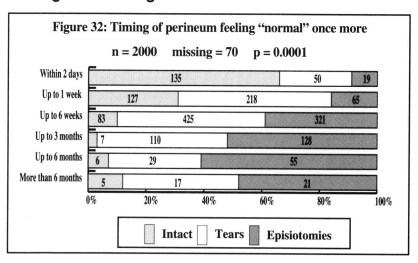

Figure 32: Timing of perineum feeling "normal" once more

n = 2000   missing = 70   p = 0.0001

	Intact	Tears	Episiotomies
Within 2 days	135	50	19
Up to 1 week	127	218	65
Up to 6 weeks	83	425	321
Up to 3 months	7	110	128
Up to 6 months	6	29	55
More than 6 months	5	17	21

56

As **Figure 32** indicates, the majority of mothers, regardless of the trauma they sustained, felt some degree of normality by the sixth week postnatally. It was the women with episiotomies and tears who needed more time before they felt they had regained "normal sensation".

Overall:

- **43% of mothers said it took up to six weeks to recover;**
- **12% said it took up to three months to recover;**
- **5% said it took up to six months;**
- **2% said it took over six months.**

109 (6%) said that they "still did not feel normal", but the length of time since these mothers had had their babies ranged from one week to twelve months.

We asked the women if they were concerned at the rate of healing and a surprisingly high number of those who answered the question (34%) said "yes", they were anxious. This number included women who actually had an intact perineum but who perhaps suffered bruising and swelling.

The percentage of women who were concerned about the rate of healing inevitably rose with the degree of trauma; just 14% of mothers with unsutured tears were anxious, as opposed to 56% of women with an episiotomy plus a tear.

"A Miracle I Ever Became Pregnant Again"

We asked the mothers about activities in their daily lives "made difficult by perineal pain". Half the mothers either said they had experienced no such difficulties, or did not fully answer the question. Of the others, the single greatest cause of difficulty was sex, 17% of mothers complained specifically of this, whereas only 3% shared the next largest complaint of not being able to sit comfortably.

The women mentioned 33 other activities which they had found difficult postnatally, including:

- walking, running, cycling, getting out of chairs;
- doing pelvic floor exercises;
- feeding, carrying and cuddling their baby.

Reading the mothers' replies we felt that the psychological problems and anxiety created by postpartum pain were often as distressing as the physical difficulties.

Here are some extracts from letters many women wrote to accompany their questionnaires:

"With my first child I could only kneel down after about ten days, and then very slowly and carefully, and not completely. Sexual intercourse has been

practically impossible, it was a miracle I ever became pregnant again."

"I sat on rubber rings and ice packs for weeks. Had to have two stitches removed by the nurse to enable me to walk to leave hospital because they were so tight. Sex was impossible for six months and depression set in. My GP - female - was helpful and organised vaginal dilators after three years of pain and "lumps" that I could still feel when I sat down in the bath. Internally on one side all nerve feeling has gone"

"Sex (resumed again after about three months) remained uncomfortable for two to three months."

"There is still tenderness and occasional discomfort after sexual intercourse. It was six months before sex was anything other than painful and yet at my postnatal (examination) I was pronounced healed."

"While I didn't have a very big tear or need many stitches I still felt as though part of my anatomy had had its shape changed and the psychological effect, as much as the physical one, made sexual intercourse difficult for some time."

It would perhaps be tempting to attribute the sexual difficulties of these and other mothers to the catch-all of psychology, were it not for the fact that a number of women found that their difficulties resolved following a subsequent birth and perineal resuturing.

A midwife gave her views:

"In three years I have had about twenty women having severe discomfort after delivery when making love. There have also been cases of women who have waited many years before they conceive again due to the perineal trauma and have had problems since their last delivery and have not known what to do - often they are dismissed by their GP as neurotic. I feel very strongly that this is a neglected area of care in the postnatal period and that no matter how good delivery technique becomes there will always be women who need extra support and care."

Neurotic?

The midwife's letter quoted from above touches on a theme tragically common to many of the accounts we were sent, the attitudes of general practitioners and other doctors. For example:

> "My doctor was most dismissive of my problems and only after I have suffered for three months was I treated."

> "I did indeed suffer for a long time afterwards - at the six week check up I literally felt like ramming my head through the wall behind me when the consultant gave me an internal. Yet he said "all was well"!.....the pain and discomfort did not subside until my daughter was ten months old."

> "I was trying to get slowly back to normal at home when I could have done with more guidance over healing problems. I don't think health visitors necessarily have the knowledge and a lot of GPs - especially the men - in my experience, can't take on board what it feels like. To them, if it looks like a tear has healed, well, then it must be alright! Not so!"

Wise Before the Event?

As we mentioned above, and in Chapter Five, many new mothers were shocked by the awful reality of perineal pain. Some women clearly felt bitter, perhaps even cheated, because they had not been adequately prepared for this aspect of their postnatal recovery:

> "I feel very strongly that women should be warned it might be many months before the perineum feels anything like "normal". I still do not feel the same..."

> "I think there should be better preparation in all antenatal classes for problems with the perineum after childbirth. I can truly say that the pain and discomfort I experienced were far worse than the experience of childbirth! I was very ignorant about what to expect and in fact did not realise that I had not been re-stitched properly until 10 weeks after the birth."

"I was surprised at how long it took the tear to heal. But even once the stitches had come out and the tear had mended I was unprepared for the length of time it took for the scar tissue to become comfortable again."

A midwife put perineal healing into perspective:

"I think it is important that women understand that perineal trauma takes time and effort to heal and I try to avoid stimulating any expectation that they should be "back to normal" too early....Sometimes it does take a while...so it is important to maintain morale. So I don't take much notice of the 28 day cut-off point (for postnatal care) in this regard. Also, scar tissue may heal up quickly initially, but then it stretches and becomes more pliable over the months to come so the whole process takes longer than women are led to expect. For example, women get told four or five days after the birth - "Oh, that's healed up nicely" when the healing process has only just begun."

Some mothers felt an alarming lack of support once they had left hospital:

"I think there is a need (for some, if not all mothers) for a Group - such as NCT - to provide some information or "help-line" on postnatal problems. Not depression or blues, but more specific medical problems which you mention in....your questionnaire...Nowhere was I able to establish whether (my set of problems) was par for the course following some births."

"I really wish I'd been warned before the birth or at least had easier access to information regarding the experiences of people with tears - problems they had and how they solved them. In other senses my husband and I were well prepared and all this aftermath has proved extremely traumatic and unexpected. It is enough to put me off having any other children and I'd be afraid the whole thing would rip apart again and I don't feel I want to repeat this very unpleasant experience! I appreciate most people don't have tears as bad as mine, but that's no consolation. I would (have) welcome(d) more support in this regard."

Stress Incontinence: Who Suffers?

"I did suffer from flatulence, incontinence and lack of control of my bowels (incredibly embarrassing) but daily post-natal exercises and that greatest healer - time - did cure me within about 16 weeks."

60

"These are the sort of problems one cannot talk about at NCT coffee mornings as they are rather delicate and personal matters."

Nearly half of the women who answered our questionnaire suffered some degree of stress incontinence.

Figure 33 compares the incidence of stress incontinence with type of perineal damage incurred.

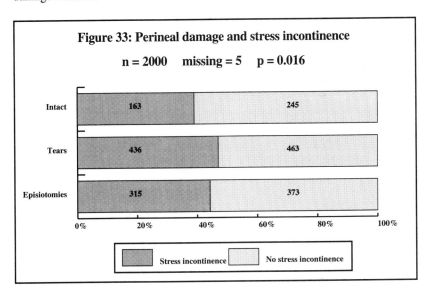

Figure 33: Perineal damage and stress incontinence

n = 2000   missing = 5   p = 0.016

Although initially slightly fewer women with an intact perineum experienced stress incontinence, we found that by six months after the birth only 3% of women were still suffering and this was not at this stage associated with the type of perineal trauma sustained at delivery.

Stress Incontinence and the Birth

In our survey, none of the following had any statistically significant effect on the incidence of stress incontinence:

● maternal age;

● parity;

● length of the first and second stages of labour;

● type of delivery - whether spontaneous or assisted by forceps or Ventouse;

● baby's birthweight.

61

We did, however, note some association between the incidence of stress incontinence and the position adopted for delivery - as **Figure 34** demonstrates.

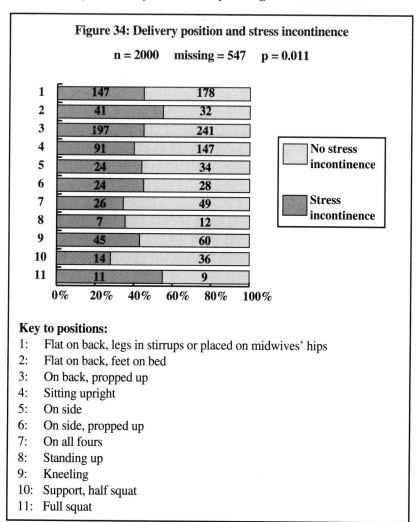

Figure 34: Delivery position and stress incontinence

n = 2000   missing = 547   p = 0.011

Key to positions:
1: Flat on back, legs in stirrups or placed on midwives' hips
2: Flat on back, feet on bed
3: On back, propped up
4: Sitting upright
5: On side
6: On side, propped up
7: On all fours
8: Standing up
9: Kneeling
10: Support, half squat
11: Full squat

We would have liked to examine the long term effect on stress incontinence of birth position but the numbers were too small to be usefully analysed.

Some women felt that their GPs were rather dismissive of the problem presented by stress incontinence. GPs may think they are justified in not being unduly concerned, since for the majority of mothers the problem does seem to resolve spontaneously by the time their babies are three months old. However, 13 weeks is a long time to be troubled in this way and for a minority of women the problem continues for considerably longer.

Control of Flatus

"Difficulty controlling flatus took me completely by surprise - it didn't last long but it was very worrying as I hadn't heard of it being a problem after childbirth - I assume it is from your question."

Over a quarter of the women reported that they had difficulty in controlling flatus postnatally, an increase of 20% over the position antenatally. We do not know whether this problem resolves in the same way that stress incontinence does, or, indeed, whether it presents a real problem to mothers.

We *did* find that:

- **women who experienced the *greatest* perineal trauma tended to have *least* difficulty controlling flatus before the birth;**
- **women who experienced the greatest perineal trauma were the *least* likely to suffer from stress incontinence before having their babies, although the *most* likely to suffer from stress incontinence *after* the birth.**

It may be that these women have particularly strong pelvic floor muscles, which do not "give" readily during childbirth, or they are less likely to relax sufficiently to facilitate a relatively untraumatic delivery of their babies. Alternatively, the observations may reflect the retrospective nature of this study where women's memories of the situation prior to birth are coloured by the situation afterwards.

A Wider Perspective

Our finding that stress incontinence is a common problem not associated with the mother's age, duration of labour, type of delivery, or degree of perineal damage is consistent with the results of a neurophysiological study. For most women having their first baby, vaginal delivery appears to cause some temporary nerve damage in the pelvic floor. For a few women serious damage may contribute to problems with continence (2).

Many women are taught pelvic floor exercises antenatally and advised to practice them frequently in order to get back to normal. Gordon and Logue (17) in a non-randomised prospective study, concluded that women taking regular exercise, such as running or swimming, fared even better than those practising pelvic floor

63

exercises. Sleep and Grant (51) in a randomised controlled trial, examined the effect of an intensive regime of pelvic floor exercises compared with a normal regime. The intense regime helped with pain but not with stress incontinence.

CHAPTER SEVEN
SUMMARY AND CONCLUSIONS

The Aims of this Study were:

1. To assess the incidence of different types of perineal trauma.
2. To determine which factors might influence the type of trauma women experience.
3. To discover what measures are taken to promote healing and relieve pain.
4. To explore the long term effects of perineal trauma.
5. To compare current practice with published research and, if a discrepancy appears, to attempt to discover why research findings are not always applied.
6. To identify areas related to perineal care worthy of clinical research of the type that the NCT cannot itself do, but midwives could.

We offer our conclusions using the format of these aims. (Percentages have been corrected to the nearest whole number for clarity; as a result, not all sums total exactly 100%).

1. Incidence of Different Types of Perineal Trauma

Our survey of 2000 women comprised of 974 first-time mothers and 1026 mothers giving birth for second or subsequent time. Most of these deliveries (88%) were attended by midwives.

- 21% of mothers had an intact perineum;
- 45% sustained tears;
- 35% had an episiotomy, some accompanied by a tear.

80% (1595) of mothers had normal (unassisted) deliveries:
- intact perineum rate of 29%;
- tear rate of 46%;
- episiotomy rate of 25%.

65

20% (403) of mothers had operative (assisted) deliveries - 16% forceps, 4% Ventouse delivery:

- intact perineum rate of 1%;
- tear rate of 28%;
- episiotomy rate of 71%.

Just under half of our survey mothers who answered the question were given *no* explanation for their tear. The main reasons given to the remaining mothers were:

1. "baby not in the best position";
2. "rapid delivery";
3. "baby too large/mother too small".

Most mothers having an *episiotomy* were given an explanation. The main reasons given were:

1. "forceps delivery";
2. "fetal distress";
3. to "speed up delivery";
4. to "avoid a tear".

380 midwives returned our questionnaire giving details of 2149 deliveries. These midwives reported an average intact perineum rate of 48%, a tear rate of 39% and an episiotomy rate of 13%. We considered these figures heartening evidence of what good midwifery care can achieve.

The main indications for performing an episiotomy according to the midwives were:

1. "fetal distress";
2. "rigid perineum";
3. "maternal distress".

We emphasise once more that both the samples in our survey were entirely self-selected and thus are not representative of all women giving birth in 1990 nor of all midwives practising at that time.

2. Factors which might Influence the Type of Trauma Women Experience

We could find *no* link between perineal damage and:
- a mother's age;
- her baby's birthweight - except in the case of premature infants;
- her baby's gestation - again, except when the baby was born prematurely;
- duration of the first stage of labour.

There *may* be a connection between a lower incidence of perineal damage and the following:
- **perineal massage during pregnancy and during delivery** - this practice may be of benefit to first-time mothers;
- **delivering standing up** - this position was associated with the best perineal outcome but, because only 22 women used this position, this finding is not conclusive;
- **delivery in water** - rates of perineal trauma were low amongst the 29 women giving birth in water, but with so few waterbirths *no firm conclusions can be made.*

There *seemed* to be a connection between perineal damage and the following:
- **parity** - the more babies a mother had delivered, the more likely she was to have had an intact perineum;
- **sharing of expectations with midwives** - most birth attendants responded positively to women's wishes and worked hard to fulfil them;
- **place of birth** - we found that, even when parity and type of delivery had been taken into account, mothers delivering their babies at home had the best chance of an intact perineum;
- **movement during the first stage of labour** - women with an intact perineum and small tears were likely to have had freedom of movement during labour;
- **rupture of the membranes** - rupture during the second stage of labour rather than earlier, whether spontaneous or artificial, was associated with a higher rate of intact perinea;
- **instructions given during delivery** - in general, the *less* instruction given by the midwife to the mother the better. The exception is a specific instruction to "relax" or "pant" during the emergence of the baby's head from the vagina;
- **expectations** - women who appeared least concerned about episiotomy prior to the birth had by far the highest episiotomy rate;

- **epidural anaesthesia** - likely to be accompanied by an episiotomy;
- **duration of the second stage** - women whose second stage of labour lasted more than 30 minutes were more likely to have an episiotomy, though this may reflect unit policy;
- **delivery position** - the worst outcome was for mothers lying flat on their backs with their legs up.

3.   Measures Taken to Promote Healing and Relieve Pain

We were pleased to note:
- nearly three-quarters of mothers requiring sutures to their perineum were attended to within 30 minutes of delivery.

We were not so pleased with other aspects of perineal repair:
- over a third of the midwives did not suture either tears or episiotomies, most said this was because they had not been given appropriate training or, having received such training were still not considered competent to suture;
- although we did not ask for details specifically, we received a number of disturbing reports of inadequate anaesthesia of the perineum prior to repair;
- only 10% of midwives suturing the perineum reported using subcuticular sutures; nearly 60% preferred an interrupted suture technique;
- over 40% of the midwives still used catgut suture material; polyglycolic sutures such as Dexon or Vicryl were used by only 13%.

After the event:

Nearly half of the mothers with episiotomies had "definite discomfort", and the same proportion of women with episiotomies *and* tears "suffered pain". In spite of this it seemed that a significant number of women turned down the offer of oral analgesia.

84% of the midwives regarded perineal pain as a "major problem" for mothers. A wide variety of "conventional" and "alternative" remedies were reported by both midwives and mothers.

From arnica to witch hazel:

Treatments for the perineum were, in descending order of popularity:
- ice packs;
- salt baths;

- physiotherapy;
- arnica;
- witch hazel.

Most midwives (82%) offered a "conventional" range of remedies, the above items plus:
- oral analgesia;
- anaesthetic gels;
- Epifoam;
- bathing and washing in general.

10% of midwives used an "alternative" approach and their remedies included:
- arnica;
- calendula;
- hypericum;
- comfrey;
- lavender oil;

plus some "conventional" remedies.

Treatments which mothers found to be the best at *relieving pain:*

thermal treatments - *warm* water in some form (bath, shower or bidet), or some kind of *cold* application (ice packs, frozen witch hazel pads, ice cold Milton-soaked pads and cold showers);

oral analgesia - 18% of women thought that oral analgesia gave the greatest relief from pain; paracetamol was considered the most effective drug on offer;

topical applications - less than a tenth of mothers felt that locally applied remedies helped the most;

mechanical relief - just a few mothers mentioned sitting on rubber rings and cushions.

Treatments which mothers found to be best at *promoting healing:*

A third of mothers agreed that regular washing of the area helped; many favouring the traditional salt bath. "Time" was the best healer for about a tenth of mothers, and arnica and various lotions were also mentioned.

Perineal wound infections were reported by 157 of the 2000 mothers:

The risk of infection increased with the degree of perineal damage incurred - small tear 1%: episiotomy and tear 22%.

Washing, generally in salty solutions, was common advice given to new mothers with perineal trauma. Nearly all of the midwives in our survey (93%) said that they gave such advice to mothers, although only 53% of *mothers* remembered being given any specific advice on perineal hygiene.

4.   The Long Term Effects of Perineal Trauma

Over a third of mothers needed six weeks for their perineum to feel "normal" again, and 2% said it took over six months. A third of all mothers told us their perineum caused them anxiety postnatally. Some women clearly felt bitter, perhaps even cheated, because they had not been adequately prepared for this aspect of their postnatal recovery:

Sexual intercourse following perineal trauma was difficult for 17% of the mothers; we received many distressing descriptive accounts of this particular problem.

Nearly half of the women who answered our questionnaire suffered some degree of stress incontinence.

The incidence of stress incontinence did not appear to be related to:
- mother's age;
- parity;
- duration of labour;
- type of delivery, whether assisted or spontaneous;
- baby's birthweight.

One factor appeared to be connected with the incidence of stress incontinence:

Women who delivered their babies "flat on their backs" or in a "full squat" were most likely to suffer from stress incontinence. The lowest incidence was associated with the "supported half squat" position.

Over a quarter of the mothers reported that they had difficulty in controlling flatus postnatally, but we did not discover the degree nor duration of this problem.

5. Comparison of Current Practice with Published Research

We learnt of several practices which were continued by midwives in spite of published research findings to the contrary.

About half the midwife sample reported that they did **not infiltrate the perineum** with either normal saline or local anaesthetic prior to suturing when there was already an epidural providing effective anaesthesia.

Nearly two-thirds of suturing midwives reported a preference for **interrupted sutures** to repair the perineum. Many midwives simply said they had been taught no other method; other reasons given tended to be somewhat muddled.

Relatively few midwives used polyglycolic acid sutures. In this instance, midwives tended to cite "hospital policy" or state that **catgut sutures** were "the only ones available".

In spite of research evidence that these practices may actually cause harm and delay healing, we were repeatedly told of:

- **Eusol** being used to clean perineal wounds;
- **ice packs** being applied to the perineum later than 24 hours following delivery;
- women being advised to sit on **rubber rings** supposedly to relieve pressure.

Taking **"salt baths"** seemed to be universally suggested to mothers with a sore or damaged perineum, in spite of firm evidence that this practice is of no demonstrable benefit. Likewise many women were asked to **dry their perineum with a hairdryer**, although there is no evidence that this is beneficial or even safe.

We could only conclude, in these instances, that midwives are not familiar with the relevant research, or, even if they *have* read the studies, prefer for their own reasons to adhere to traditional practices.

6. Research Potentials

This report describes a number of factors which are associated with the degree of perineal trauma that women experience during childbirth. Because these factors were identified in a retrospective study, none of them can be assumed to cause or prevent perineal trauma.

71

Throughout this study we have been very aware of the complexities of factors which affect perineal outcome. For example, individual features of labour, such as preservation of the membranes, and freedom of movement, are generally, but by no means exclusively, part of a "package" of inter-related factors which each contribute to the type of labour and delivery experienced. A mother who remains upright and mobile during her labour is less likely to require oxytocic drugs to augment her contractions (49) and is thus more likely to avoid continual fetal monitoring and strong analgesic drugs. On the other hand, a women whose blood pressure is high may be advised to have epidural anaesthesia during labour, and this one action will limit movement, probably necessitate internal fetal monitoring (and thus rupture of the membranes) and perhaps affect the type of delivery. These simple examples indicate in part why it has not been possible to identify the effect of some individual factors in this study.

We would therefore like to see prospective studies address the issue of preventing perineal trauma. For instance:

● Do women's views during pregnancy influence the perineal trauma they experience during childbirth?

In addition, randomised controlled trials could answer questions such as:

● If women are given the opportunity to try out a wide range of positions which might be comfortable during labour and delivery do they experience less perineal trauma than women whose antenatal classes are more passive?

● Do labours characterised by early artificial rupture of membranes (and possibly syntocinon infusions) lead to more perineal trauma compared to unmanaged labours?

● If women are given no instructions during the second stage of labour except to "pant" or "relax" at the crowning of their baby's head, do they experience less perineal trauma than women given specific encouragement to push?

● Does antenatal perineal massage reduce the perineal trauma for women expecting their first baby?

● Can encouraging women to share their views with midwives help mothers to fulfil their expectations of perineal care?

- Does labouring and possibly giving birth in water affect perineal outcome?

It is possible that contributory factors are able to affect the perineum significantly only if they appear coincidentally with other factors. For example, if a woman's views during pregnancy influence her experience at childbirth, surely this causal relationship is tempered by the willingness of midwives to encourage her to express her views? Likewise, is the effect of a woman's position at delivery on perineal outcome in turn influenced by the instructions she is given by her midwife? The possibility of factors working together, or in competition, must be recognised.

Observational studies could also provide valuable information:
- The practice of midwives whose clients generally give birth with minimal perineal trauma could be observed to identify the factors most likely to lead to childbirth with an intact perineum.

The designers of all these studies must bear in mind that it is not only whether a perineum is cut or tears that is important to a woman - but her subsequent comfort and wellbeing and the effect on her relationship with her baby and partner. Since the techniques and materials used to repair perineal trauma, and the subsequent care and treatment of the area have a bearing on these features of a woman's life, it is vital that outstanding questions are answered:

- Comparisons between Dexon (a polyglycolic acid suture) and catgut have been thorough but there is now an unproven assumption that Vicryl (another polyglycolic acid suture) is as good as Dexon. Is this true?

- The research findings on cold therapy are confused but it remains a popular remedy for the traumatised perineum: is cold therapy appropriate?

- Arnica, a homoeopathic remedy, was very widely used and highly regarded by the mothers in our survey: how effective is it and does it have any side effects?

- The contribution of pelvic floor exercises and, indeed, other forms of physical activity to long term physical recovery is not fully understood: how can women best help themselves?

More fundamentally:

Research findings concerning glycerol impregnated catgut were largely ignored. Epifoam and Eusol were still used in spite of evidence that these substances are potentially harmful. The benefits of Ventouse delivery over forceps delivery do not appear to have been widely recognised. *How may health professionals be encouraged to abandon treatments which have been shown to be detrimental to health?*

Health professionals who wish to check whether the care they offer is supported by rigorous research studies can refer to the *Cochrane Collaboration Pregnancy and Childbirth Database* (13). This database collates the results of randomised controlled trials from around the world and is updated every six months. Ongoing and completed projects are also recorded on two databases at the National Perinatal Epidemiological Unit (NPEU), Radcliffe Infirmary, Oxford, OX2 6HE, the *International Register of Perinatal Trials* (40) and the *Midwifery Research Database (MIRIAD)* (41).

The *Midwives' Information and Resource Service (MIDIRS)* offers invaluable assistance to health professionals and others wishing to keep up with current practice and thinking. MIDIRS publishes a quarterly *Midwifery Digest* (37) of recent papers and publications of interest to midwives, and their Midwifery Database (36) can be used to produce literature searches of specific topics.

Finally, health professionals motivated to test methods of care for themselves can turn to the Perinatal Trials Service at the NPEU which offers the skills and resources to assist research groups in the design and implementation of clinical trials.

CHAPTER EIGHT

RECOMMENDATIONS

To Health Workers

To NCT Workers and Supporters

To Childbearing Women

To Labour Companions and Partners

The National Childbirth Trust recommends the following:

To Health Workers -

1. We recommend that both individual midwives, and maternity units as a whole, **monitor their perineal injury rates** carefully and review them regularly, with a view to increasing the number of intact perinea and reducing the degree of perineal pain. We feel that individual midwives can learn much from each other's experiences and that these should be shared in a supportive and non-judgemental fashion.

2. We would like to see **women more realistically prepared** for pain and other perineal-related problems - including wound infection, stress incontinence and painful sexual intercourse - which they may experience after the birth of their babies. We appreciate that this may be difficult to do without appearing to be rather negative about the outcome of labour, but we do feel that information sensitively given in the antenatal clinic or classroom will help to alleviate the shock so many new mothers experience as the "harsh reality" hits them. The special communication needs of women who have difficulty with hearing or reading and those whose first language is not English should be remembered.

3. We hope to see a further strengthening of the present trend for women and midwives to work in **informed partnership** during delivery to ensure the best possible outcome, physically and emotionally, for mothers and their babies. Mutual sharing of information and expectations is intrinsic to this partnership, and such communication is optimised when there is **continuity of midwifery carer**, *ideally* throughout the childbearing period but *critically* during labour.

4. We trust that all women will continue to be enabled and encouraged to move

about freely during labour, and to **adopt positions in which they feel comfortable** when delivering their babies. Since the environment for both these recommendations is optimised when the labour is conducted in the mother's own home, we recommend that women who choose to give birth at home are given support.

5. We recommend that all women who require perineal repair following delivery are **sutured by the professional most appropriate** for their individual circumstances. In many, if not most, instances this will be the midwife who assisted with the delivery of the baby. We therefore trust that **all midwives will be trained** to fulfil this aspect of their professional role.

6. We strongly recommend that when suturing is necessary **sufficient and appropriate anaesthesia** is given to ensure a painless experience.

7. We further *strongly* recommend that **suturing materials and techniques** chosen for the repair of damaged perinea are the most appropriate in the light of available research.

8. We recommend that mothers are reassured (as far as possible in the light of currently available evidence) about the **safety of suitable oral analgesia when breastfeeding** and encouraged to take advantage of these drugs if required to relieve perineal pain postnatally.

9. We would like to see new mothers given **clear and specific instructions on perineal hygiene.** These instructions should be based on current research findings and could be usefully reinforced by graphical posters displayed in toilets and bathrooms. Posters should be designed with the needs of non-English speaking women in mind and audiocassettes should be available for the visually impaired.

10. We would like all health workers to ensure the maintenance/attainment of **high standards of cleanliness in hospital bathrooms and toilets**. We further suggest that methods of **monitoring levels of postnatal infections** be investigated, as recommended by the Winterton report (25).

11. We strongly recommend that only remedies and therapies which have been shown **by sound research** to be of benefit are routinely used to treat sore or infected perinea. We emphasise that this recommendation applies equally to

"alternative" and "conventional" treatments. To this end, we trust that encouragement and finance will increasingly be made available for appropriate research projects.

12. We sincerely hope that women who are troubled postnatally by stress incontinence or painful intercourse are dealt with **sympathetically and respectfully** by *all* health workers. Severe postpartum perineal pain and incontinence, whether of urine, flatus or faeces, should not be allowed to fall into the "things will get better" category of professional attention; the distress of these women should be recognised. We therefore trust that health workers will offer appropriate reassurance and information based on current research findings and will readily refer women to specialist professional help when indicated.

To NCT Workers and Supporters -

1. We recommend that **antenatal teachers** incorporate into their classes information on the factors which appear to minimise perineal damage at delivery. We feel it is also very important that women are offered research-based guidance on possible perineal problems postnatally: their prevention, alleviation and cure, plus some suggestions as to when normality becomes abnormality and professional help is required.

2. We hope that **postnatal supporters and "baby group" facilitators** will bear in mind that some postnatal problems are "the sort that one cannot talk about at NCT coffee mornings, as they are rather delicate and personal...." (to quote one survey mother) - but it is often precisely these problems which cause the greatest private distress and pain. Mothers can help other mothers by being alert to cues that all is not well and by demonstrating a readiness to listen constructively. Some postnatal supporters will also be able to offer specific information if required, for example, on local health facilities and support groups.

3. We urge **breastfeeding counsellors** to remember how potentially disruptive and distracting perineal problems can be to breastfeeding mothers and babies.

4. All NCT members should encourage **sound, appropriate and ethical research** into the prevention, alleviation and treatment of perineal trauma.

To Childbearing Women -
For the birth of your baby:

1. **Understand that research is ongoing** and that you will be making some decisions about the birth of your baby on the basis of incomplete evidence.

2. **Bear in mind that this report alone cannot tell you how to minimise perineal trauma.** Our survey was essentially a descriptive study of past events and our findings are not statistically applicable to the wider population of childbearing women. We simply offer ideas and suggestions arising out of the experiences of a defined group of women.

3. **Make your wishes regarding perineal care clear** to your midwife. Remember that those women in our study who wished to avoid both an episiotomy and a tear, and those who expressed these wishes to their midwives, were the women who experienced least trauma. Randomised controlled trials show that reducing the episiotomy rate also, to some extent, increases the intact perineum rate.

4. **Ask your midwife how often she performs episiotomies.** Randomised controlled trials show that women delivered by midwives with the lowest episiotomy rates are more likely to have an intact perineum.

5. **Antenatal perineal massage might help** to reduce perineal trauma at the birth of your first baby.

Postnatal hygiene and comfort:

6. **If you need stitching after you have had your baby, ask for pain relief** if it is not offered and request that your attendant waits until the anaesthetic is fully effective before starting to stitch. Ask for more pain relief if it is needed.

7. **It is important to wash your perineum carefully** and this may be difficult when it is sore. Whether using a bidet, a hand-held shower attachment or a jug of water, the flow of water must be directed from the front to the back of the area to minimise the risk of washing faecal material from the anus onto the perineum.

8. **It is important to dry your perineum thoroughly** since infection is more likely to occur in damp, soggy skin. Dabbing your perineum dry with a pad of soft toilet paper is probably the most effective way to dry the area. The use of hairdryers for drying the perineum is not recommended; firstly, because a hairdryer is itself a potential source of infection in this situation, and secondly because excessive drying may inhibit healing.

9. **Sanitary towels should be held snugly in place** so that they do not rub against the wound when you are walking.

10. **If it is uncomfortable sitting to feed your baby, try lying down** with him or her lying beside you. Alternatively, you could try sitting on a Valley Cushion - ask your NCT antenatal teacher or postnatal supporter for details.

11. **Constipation can be avoided** with a well balanced diet including plenty of fruit, vegetables and bran - and a drink whenever thirsty. It is quite normal for a few days to go by after delivery before you feel ready to pass a bowel motion. Some women are worried that opening their bowels in the early days will be painful or will cause further damage to their perineum - the latter is normally extremely unlikely. Holding a thick pad of toilet paper or a clean sanitary towel against your perineum when passing a motion may help you feel more comfortable. If your perineal wound is extensive and involves the anus your midwife will probably offer additional advice.

12. **Haemorrhoids ("piles")** after childbirth can be painful but are usually a short term problem. Many women assume that all postpartum pain in the perineal area is due to a tear or episiotomy wound, whereas for some women much of the discomfort is caused by protruding haemorrhoids, easily felt as soft lumps in the anal area. The discomfort of haemorrhoids can be eased by thoroughly lubricating the anal area and gently pushing haemorrhoids back inside the anus with your fingers. Medicated creams to relieve the pain and swelling of haemorrhoids are readily available from your midwife, GP or pharmacy.

13. **Vaginal dryness** is a common but temporary experience caused by the hormones of breastfeeding. Some women find that using a lubricant such as K-Y Jelly around the vaginal opening can help relaxation and penetration when first resuming sexual intercourse. Gentle perineal massage during foreplay to explore any tender areas may also help.

14. **Evaluation of maternity services is very important.** You can influence developments in maternity care by praising what you find good and by suggesting improvements. You may be invited to comment as part of a consumer satisfaction audit. If not, you may wish to write a personal letter to managers and individuals involved in your care to identify features of your care which are of particular importance to you, highlighting excellence or focussing attention where there is room for improvement. If you are not satisfied with your care at any stage, or with the response to your initial communication on the subject, you can seek advice from your local Community Health Council, the local branch of the NCT or a pressure group such as the Association for Improvements in Maternity Services (AIMS).

15. **Research is vital for good maternity care**. We hope parents will give their *informed* consideration to invitations to participate in worthwhile research. Furthermore, rather than simply accepting or rejecting the research projects offered by health professionals, scientists or drug companies you may wish to influence how research is conducted, or indeed what research is undertaken. The NCT aims to represent women and their families so that what they have to say about their experiences is no longer "ignored, forgotten or dismissed..(but) publicised and specifically drawn to the attention of health professionals, policy makers and researchers" (39). You are invited to send any suggestions for maternity care research to the NCT Research and Information Group.

To Labour Companions and Partners —

1. **Find out in advance** the wishes of the woman you are supporting and help her to communicate them to her birth attendants.

2. **Continue to support** the woman you are with throughout the stitching rather than just cuddling the baby. Remember that careful repair of any perineal injury is vital. Ensure that she has sufficient pain relief should she need stitching.

3. Realise **that it may take a long time for a woman to get "back to normal".** Enthusiasm for a sexual relationship may be reduced for weeks or months by discomfort, exhaustion or simply total absorption in her new baby.

4. **Help your partner to get the care she needs** from the health professionals if she is suffering pain or discomfort or other abnormal symptoms soon after the

birth or any time later. Some women find that the most appropriate treatment, information and support by requesting to see an obstetric physiotherapist.

NCT leaflets to use:

Caring for your pelvic floor London: National Childbirth Trust, 1988
Sex in pregnancy and after childbirth London: National Childbirth Trust, 1988

These, and many other publications of interest to parents and professionals, are available from:
NCT (Maternity Sales) Ltd, 239 Shawbridge Street, Glasgow, G42 1QN. Tel: 0141-636 0600

**There are NCT branches throughout the country which offer antenatal classes, breast feeding counselling and postnatal support.
For information about your local branch contact:
NCT, Alexandra House, Oldham Terrace, London W3 6NH
Tel: 0181 - 992 8637**

Women and Research: A Postscript from the Research and Information Group of the NCT, September 1993.

While we were collating and analysing the individual experiences of 2000 women and 380 midwives, the House of Commons Select Committee on Health was listening to women and health professionals describe how maternity care is offered to all childbearing women.

Amongst many recommendations, the Committee's report (known as the Winterton Report, 25) proposed that women be treated as "equal partners" with their carers in decision making, and that new methods of care be "rigorously evaluated". We would like to see these two proposals drawn together to bring women into the research process as equal partners with professionals.

In answering our questionnaire women identified health problems which seriously affect their lives. In conversations with their midwives women daily identify those areas in which they wish to be well informed. Through a consideration of both their personal health and the questions which remain for them unanswered, women can list their research priorities.

We would expect greater success in identifying measures of client satisfaction, as recommended in the Winterton Report (25), if maternity service users were full collaborators in the research process, from setting the research agenda and planning and conducting research projects, to implementing research findings.

"Too many fashionable interventions in intrapartum care have been introduced without evaluation either of cost-benefit ratios or the reactions of women who undergo them" (25). The Winterton report recommends that all new developments be "rigorously evaluated" against a wide range of criteria including the satisfaction of women and their families and the long and the short term health of mothers and their babies (25). We would like to extend these recommendations to cover all forms of care during pregnancy, birth and afterwards, so that all are adequately investigated for their benefits, risks and side-effects.

We further believe that effort should not be merely focussed on reducing the worst effects of poor heath or inappropriate care but also be directed towards the nurturing of normal, physiological pregnancy and birth. Such research should encompass not only the immediate physical safety and long term health of childbearing women and their families, but should include appropriate social and emotional aspects of their total wellbeing.

REFERENCES

1.   Alexander, J., Levy, V. and Roch, S. 1990: *Postnatal Care.* Macmillan, London.

2.   Allen, R.E., Hosker, G.L., Smith, A.R.B. and Warrel 1990: Pelvic floor damage and childbirth: a neurophysiological study. *British Journal of Obstetrics and Gynaecology* 97:9, 770-779.

3.   Anon. 1990: Cutting Edge. *Mother and Baby* October. 42-46.

4.   Avery, M.D. and Burket, B.A. 1986: Perineal massage: effect on the incidence of episiotomy and laceration in a nurse-midwifery service. *Journal of Nurse-Midwifery* 32:3, 128-134.

5.   Avery, M.D. and Van Arsdale, L. 1987: Perineal massage: effect on the incidence of episiotomy and perineal laceration in a nulliparous population. *Journal of Nurse-Midwifery* 32:3, 181-184.

6.   Ayliffe, G.A.B., Babb, J.R., Collins, J., Deverill, C. and Varney, J. 1975: Disinfection of baths and bathwater. *Nursing Times* 71:37, "Contact" supplement no. 3, 22-23.

7.   Bartlett, R. 1989: Episiotomy - have you been stitched up? *Mother.* November, 20-21.

8.   Borton, H. and Newburn, M. 1989: *Rupture of Membranes in Labour.* The National Childbirth Trust, London.

9.   British Medical Association and the Royal Pharmaceutical Society of Great Britain, 1992: *British National Formulary.* No. 24. London.

10.   Burns, E. and Greenish, K. 1993: Pooling information. *Nursing Times* 89:8, 47-49.

11.   Caldeyro-Barcia, R. 1979: The influence of maternal bearing-down efforts during the second stage on fetal wellbeing. *Birth and Family* 6:1, 17-21.

12.   Caddow, P. (Ed.) 1989: Applied Microbiology. Scutari, London.

13.   Cochrane Collaboration Pregnancy and Childbirth Database available from Cochrane Updates on Disk, Update Software Ltd., Manor Cottage, Little Milton, Oxford, OX44 7QB.

14.   Cocks, P. 1986: Preparation of the perineum for normal childbirth, *Special Delivery* June, 4-7. Childbirth Educators Association.

15.   Dunn, P. 1983: Squatting, *New Generation* 2:1, 2

16.   Gibson, J., Haslam, Y., Laurenson, L. *et al.* 1991: Double blind trial of Arnica in acute trauma patients. *British Homoeopathy Research Group Communications* no. 21.

17.   Gordon, H. and Logue, M. 1985: Perineal muscle function after childbirth. *Lancet* ii, 20th July, 123-135.

18.   Grant, A. 1989: Repair of perineal trauma after childbirth. In: Chalmers, I., Enkin, M. and Keirse, M. (Eds.). *Effective Care in Pregnancy and Childbirth,* 1170-81. Oxford University Press, Oxford.

19.   Grant, A., Sleep, J., Ashurst, H. and Spencer, J. 1989: Dyspareunia associated with the use of glycerol-impregnated catgut to repair perineal trauma, report of
a three year follow up study. *British Journal of Obstetrics and Gynaecology* 96:6,
741-743.
20.   Grant, A., Sleep, J., McIntosh, J. and Ashurst, H. 1989: Ultrasound and pulsed
electromagnetic energy treatment for perineal trauma: a randomised placebo-controlled
trial. *British Journal of Obstetrics and Gynaecology* 96:4, 434-439.
21.   Greer, I.A. and Cameron, A.D. 1984: Topical pramoxine and hydrocortisone
foam versus placebo in relief of post partum episiotomy symptoms and wound
healing. *Scottish Medical Journal* 29, 104-106.
22.   Greenshields, W. 1988: *Postnatal Infection.* The National Childbirth Trust,
London.
23.   Harris, M. 1992: The impact of research findings on current practice in
relieving postpartum perineal pain in a large district hospital. *Midwifery* 8:3, 125-
131.
24.   Hofmeyer, G.J., Piccioni, V. and Blauhof, P. 1990: Postpartum homoeopathic
Arnica montana: a potency-finding pilot study. *British Journal of Clinical Practice*
44:12, 619-621.
25.   *House of Commons Select Committee on Health's Report on Maternity
Services* 1992. (Number 430-I: £19.40) Available from HMSO, PO Box 276,
London SW8 5DT (071-873 9090).
26.   Johnson, A. 1987: Wound healing under a microscope. *Community
Outlook,* January, 12-15.
27.   Johnson, A. 1988: The cleansing ethic. *Community Outlook*, February 9-10.
28.   Johnson, A. 1988: Wound management: "Are you getting it right?". *Professional Nurse* 3:8, 306-308.
29.   Khan, G.Q. and Lilford, R.J. 1987: Wound pain may be reduced by prior
infiltration of the episiotomy site after delivery under epidural anaesthesia. *British
Journal of Obstetrics and Gynaecology* 94: 4, April, 341-344.
30.   Kitzinger, S. and Simkin, P. 1986: *Episiotomy and the Second Stage of
Labour.* Pennypress, Seattle, U.S.A.
31.   Kitzinger, S. and Walters, R. 1981: *Some Women's Experiences of
Episiotomy.* The National Childbirth Trust, London.
32.   Logue, M. 1991: Putting research into practice: perineal management during
delivery. In: Robinson, S. and Thomson, A.M. (Eds.) *Midwives Research and
Childbirth* Volume 2, chapter 9, 252-270. Chapman and Hall, London
33.   Lowthian, P. 1985: A sore point. *Nursing Mirror* 161:9, 30-32.
34.   MacFarlane, A. and Mugford, M. 1984: *Birth Counts: Statistics of pregnancy and childbirth.* HMSO London
35.   Maxwell, L. 1992: Therapeutic use of ultrasound. *Physiotherapy* 78:6, 421-
426.

36. Midwives Information and Resource Service, MIDIRS Midwifery Database at MIDIRS, 9 Elmdale Road, Bristol, BS8 1SL.

37. Midwives Information and Resource Service, MIDIRS Midwifery Digest, available from MIDIRS, 9 Elmdale Road, Bristol, BS8 1SL.

38. Moore, W. and James, D.K. 1989: A random trial of three topical analgesic agents in the treatment of episiotomy pain following instrumental delivery. *Journal of Obstetrics and Gynaecology* 10: 1, 35-39.

39. Moran-Ellis, J. 1991: Rupture of Membranes in Labour. *Journal of Obstetrics and Gynaecology* 11 (supplement 1), S6-S10.

40. National Perinatal Epidemiology Unit. *International Register of Perinatal Trials*. NPEU, Radcliffe Infirmary, Oxford, OX2 6HE.

41. National Perinatal Epidemiology Unit. *Midwifery Research Database (MIRIAD)*. NPEU, Radcliffe Infirmary, Oxford, OX2 6HE.

42. Parnell, C., Langhoff-Roos, J., Iversen, R. and Damgaard, P. 1993: Pushing method in the expulsive phase of labor, a randomised trial. *Acta Obstet. Gynaecol. Scand.* 72: 31-35.

43. Pusey, J., Hodge, C., Wilkinson, P. and Johanson, R. 1991: Maternal Impressions of Forceps or Silc-cup. *British Journal of Obstetrics and Gynaecology* 98:5, 487-488.

44. Renfrew, M. and Hanna, W. 1993: A Literature Review of Management of the Perineum at Delivery. Unpublished. NPEU, Radcliffe Infirmary, Oxford, OX2 6HE.

45. Research and Information Group, NCT, 1990: Perineum in childbirth, *New Generation*, 9:4, Insert.

46. Research and Information Group, NCT, 1989: Postnatal recovery questionnaire, *New Generation*, 8:2, Insert. (Report in preparation)

47. Research and Information Group, NCT 1991: The National Childbirth Trust, *Midwives' Chronicle and Nursing Notes*, 104:1237, 57-58.

48. Rhode, M.A. and Barger, M.K. 1990: Perineal care, then and now. *Journal of Nurse-Midwifery* 35:4, 220-230.

49. Roberts, J. 1989: Maternal position during the first stage of labour. In: Chalmers, I., Enkin, M. and Keirse, M. (Eds.). *Effective Care in Pregnancy and Childbirth*, 883-892. Oxford University Press, Oxford.

50. Sleep, J. 1990: Postnatal perineal care. In: Alexander, J., Levy, V. and Roch, S. (Eds). *Postnatal care*. MacMillan, London.

51. Sleep, J. and Grant, A. 1987: Pelvic floor exercise in postnatal care - the report of a randomised controlled trial to compare an intensive regime with the programme in current use. *Midwifery* 3:4, 158-164.

52. Sleep, J. and Grant, A. 1987: West Berkshire Perineal Management Trial, three year follow up. *British Medical Journal* 295, 26th Sept., 749-751.

53.   Sleep, J., Grant, A., Garcia, J., Elbourne, D., Spencer, J. and Chalmers, I. 1984: West Berkshire Perineal Management Trial. *British Medical Journal* 289, 8th September, 587-590.

54.   Sleep, J., Roberts, J. and Chalmers, I. 1989: Care during the second stage of labour, In: Chalmers, I., Enkin, M. and Keirse, M. (Eds.). *Effective Care in Pregnancy and Childbirth,* 1129-44. Oxford University Press, Oxford.

55.   Spellacy, W. 1965: A double-blind controlled study of a medicated pad for relief of episiotomy pain. *American Journal of Obstetrics and Gynecology* 92, 15 May 272.

56.   Spencer, J., Grant, A., Elbourne, D., Garcia, J. and Sleep, J. 1986: A randomized comparison of glycerol-impregnated chromic catgut with untreated chromic catgut for repair of perineal trauma. *British Journal of Obstetrics and Gynaecology* 93:5, 426-440.

57.   Thompson, D.J., 1987: No episiotomy?! *Australian and New Zealand Journal of Obstetrics and Gynaecology* February 27 (1), 18-20.

58.   UKCC, 1991: *Handbook of Midwives' Rules.* London.

59.   UKCC, 1991: *A Midwife's Code of Conduct.* London.

60.   Vacca, A. and Keirse, M. 1989: Instrumental vaginal deliveries. In: Chalmers, I., Enkin, M. and Keirse, M. (Eds.). *Effective Care in Pregnancy and Childbirth.* 1216-1233. Oxford University Press, Oxford.

61.   Warren, C. and Kargar, I. 1992: Decision time for midwives. *Nursing Times* 88, 26-28.

62.   Yearwood, J. 1991: The valley cushion. *Midwives' Chronicle and Nursing Notes* 104:1246, 336.

GLOSSARY

Amniotic membranes - the thin-walled bag, containing fluid, which surrounds the baby during pregnancy.

Crowning - the term used to describe the situation when the largest diameter of the baby's head is present at the vaginal outlet.

Epidural - an injection, or infusion, of anaesthetic into the epidural space around the spinal column.

Episiotomy - a cut made into the perineum to enlarge the vaginal outlet.

Fetus - the baby from 10 weeks gestation to birth.

Flatus - gas or air in the bowel or stomach.

Gestation - the age of the fetus (in weeks) from the last menstrual period.

Haematoma - a collection of blood trapped in the tissues.

Interrupted sutures - a method of stitching tissue where each stitch is inserted separately and is not connected to the adjoining stitches.

Introitus - the entrance to the vagina.

Multiparous - a pregnant woman who has delivered a baby before.

Oedema - the collection of extra fluid in body tissues.

Parity - the number of pregnancies a woman has carried.

Perineum - the area between the entrance to the vagina and the anus (back passage).

Primaparous - a woman pregnant for the first time.

Pudendal block - an injection of local anaesthetic into the pudendal nerve.

Pulsed electro-magnetic therapy - treatment with electrical impulses to reduce swelling and promote healing.

Randomised controlled trial - a study comparing the outcomes of two or more groups (receiving different treatments or forms of care) to which individuals are allocated at random (i.e. by chance).

Spinal block - an injection of anaesthetic into the spinal column.

Subcuticular sutures - a continuous running stitch placed below the surface of the skin.

Stress incontinence - the involuntary leakage of urine, often associated with coughing, sneezing or exertion.

Ultrasound therapy - treatment with sound waves to reduce swelling and promote healing.

Vacuum extraction - a technique for assisting the delivery of the baby using a suction apparatus (Ventouse delivery).

Vasoconstriction - narrowing of the blood vessels.

The Perineum in Childbirth

The Research and Information Group of the National Childbirth Trust is currently enquiring into perineal trauma in childbirth. If you gave birth in 1990 we would be glad to receive this questionnaire completed by you by **February 28th, 1991.**
We would like to hear from women who had an intact perineum as well as those who had a tear or episiotomy.
We would find it useful to have your name and address but please feel free to remain anonymous. Mother's comments may be used anonymously in the published report of the survey. This questionnaire may be photocopied and distributed to non-NCT members, or if time allows, published in local NCT newsletters.
Please answer each question by putting relevant number in each box, or X when question is not applicable.

ABOUT YOU AND YOUR BABY
Name .... Age ....
Address ....
Hospital ....
NCT BRANCH (if NCT member) ....
Baby's age now .... Baby's weight at birth ....
Your occupation (current or prior to having family) ....

1. Was this your first or a subsequent baby? (Enter 1,2,3, etc. and add TW for twins. □
2. How many weeks pregnant were you when your baby was born? □ □
3. Where did you have your baby? (1) Home (2) GP Unit (3) Consultant Unit (4) Elsewhere □
4. Where had you intended to have your baby? (1) Home (2) GP Unit (3) Consultant Unit (4) Elsewhere □
5. How many days did you spend in hospital? □ □
6. Did you have any particular views on tears and episiotomies before the birth? (1) Yes (2) No (If yes, please state briefly) □

....

7. Were you able to discuss your views on tears and episiotomies with the midwife or doctor before the birth? (1) Yes (2) No □

LABOUR

8. During labour, did you have freedom of movement and position: ☐
   (1) At all times (2) Most of the time (3) Only for a short time.
9. Did you have an epidural? (1) Yes (2) No. ☐
10. Were your membranes ruptured (1) spontaneously ☐
    (2) artificially (3) both?
11. Did the rupture of membranes occur during (1) the first stage of labour ☐
    (2) the second stage of labour?
12. What position did you adopt for delivery? (1) Flat on back,
    legs in stirrups, or placed on midwives' hips (2) Flat on back, feet
    on bed (3) On back, propped up (4) Sitting upright (5) On side
    (6) On side, propped up (7) On all fours (8) Standing up
    (9) Kneeling (10) Support, half squat (11) Full squat. ☐ ☐
13. Did you spend any part of your labour in a birthing pool or bath?
    (1) Yes (2) No ☐
14. If YES, how long did you spend in the water in total?.............
15. Was the baby born while you were in the water? (1) Yes (2) No ☐
16. How many hours did the first stage of labour last? ☐ ☐
17. For how long were you pushing the baby out?...........................minutes.
18. When the cervix was fully dilated, were you encouraged: ☐
    (1) to start pushing (2) not to push until you wanted to
    (3) no instruction given.
19. Were you encouraged: (1) to push long and hard for as ☐
    long as the contraction lasted (2) to push in short bursts
    (3) no instruction given.
20. Were you encouraged (1) to hold your breath while pushing ☐
    (2) breathe softly (3) no instruction given
21. When the head was crowning, were you encouraged: ☐
    (1) to keep pushing (2) to pant (3) to relax (4) no instruction given
22. What kind of delivery did you have? (1) Normal (2) Forceps ☐
    (3) Caesarean (4) Vacuum extraction
23. Did you have: (1) an intact perineum (2) an unstitched tear ☐
    (3) a stitched tear (4) an episiotomy (5) an episiotomy and tear?
24. Did you have any other tears around the vaginal area, other than ☐
    of the perineum? (1) Yes (2) No
    (Please state where if you know, labia, urethra, clitoris)..................
25. Were you given any local anaesthetic into the perineum before ☐
    tearing or having an episiotomy (1) Yes (2) No (3) Don't know.
26. Did the midwife or doctor massage your perineum to help ☐
    it stretch during labour? (1) Yes (2) No (3) Don't know.
27. If your perineum was massaged during labour, was this: ☐
    (1) soothing, (2) uncomfortable (3) painful?

28. Did you practice perineal massage during pregnancy? (1) Yes (2) No. ☐

AFTER THE BIRTH

29. If you had a tear, what was the reason given to you?..............
....

30. If you had an episiotomy, what was the reason given to you?...........
....

31. If you had an episiotomy, who performed it? (1) Midwife ☐
(2) GP (3) Hospital doctor (4) Other

32. If you had a tear, who repaired it? (1) Midwife (2) GP ☐
(3) Hospital doctor (4) Other

33. If you had an episiotomy, who repaired it (1) Midwife (2) GP ☐
(3) Hospital Doctor (4) Other

34. Were you given any pain relief just before the repair? (1) Yes ☐
(2) No. Please state what you were given................................

35. How long after the birth did you have to wait for the repair to ☐
be done? .... Hours .... Minutes ....

36. Who was your **main** attendant during labour? (1) Midwife ☐
(2) GP (3) Hospital Doctor (4) Other

37. Did you have a postnatal infection occurring up to 14 days ☐ ☐
after the birth? (please put all relevant numbers if more than one) ☐ ☐
(1) No (2) Perineal stitches (3) Caesarean stitches ☐ ☐ ☐
(4) uterine (5) urinary (6) thrush (7) other

38. If this was not your first baby, did you in any previous births have: ☐
(please state the worst injury) (1) an unstitched tear
(2) a stitched tear (3) an episiotomy (4) an episiotomy and tear
(5) a tear of labia, urethra or clitoris?

39. In the first few days after birth, did your perineum cause you: ☐
(1) no discomfort (2) slight discomfort (3) definite discomfort (4) pain?

40. In the first few days after birth, did your perineum feel ☐
(1) as you expected (2) more painful than you expected (3)
less painful than you expected?

41. Was any pain relieving medicine given to you for perineal discomfort: ☐
(1) fully effective (2) partially effective (3) not effective at all.
Please state what you were given...

42. Were there any treatments applied to your perineum to relieve pain? ☐
(1) Yes (2) No. If yes, please state which. ....

43. Did you: (1) accept pain relief (2) refuse pain relief ☐
(3) had to ask for pain relief (4) were refused pain relief when you
asked for it (5) had to wait a long time for pain relief (over half an hour)
(6) other

44. If you had a perineal stitch infection, please state what treatment was given.
....
45. If your perineum was sore or infected, who gave you advice and treatment for it? Please state...
46. Did you use any remedies of your own? (1) Yes (2) No. ☐
    If yes, please state which...
47. Please state which remedy or treatment was most effective in relieving pain
....
48. Please state which remedy or treatment was most effective in healing the perineum...
49. How long was it before your perineum felt back to normal? ☐
    (1) Within two days (2) up to 1 week (3) Up to 6 weeks (4) Up to 3 months
    (5) up to 6 months (6) more than 6 months (7) still suffering.
50. If you had a tear or episiotomy, were you concerned at the ☐
    rate of healing? (1) Yes (2) No.
51. Either before or after having your baby, were you given any ☐
    particular advice on how to keep your perineum clean after the birth
    (1) Yes (2) No. If yes, please state.................................
52. Apart from immediately after your baby was born, during the rest of your ☐
    stay in hospital, were you provided with (1) sterile sanitary towels (2)
    unsterile towels (3) no towels, you had to provide your own.
53. Which sanitary towels did you buy and use either during your hospital stay
    and/or after you went home? ....
54. Would you practise perineal massage during a future pregnancy if you ☐
    thought it might help to prevent damage to your perineum? (1) Yes
    (2) Maybe (3) No
55. After having your baby, did you suffer from any stress incontinence ☐
    (leakage of urine when you cough, sneeze, or on exertion)? (1) Yes (2) No
56. If you did have stress incontinence, for how long did it last? ☐
    (1) less than six weeks (2) six weeks to 12 weeks (3) 3 to 6 months
    (4) more than six months (5) still suffering
57. Did you suffer from stress incontinence **before** having your baby? ☐
    (1) Yes (2) No
58. Since having your baby, have you had any difficulty controlling flatus ☐
    (wind), or your bowels? (1) Yes (2) No
59. Did you have any difficulty controlling flatus or your bowels before ☐
    you had your baby? (1) Yes (2) No
60. Which activities did you consider were, or still are, made difficult by ☐
    perineal pain?..

Please feel free to add comments, using a separate sheet of paper if necessary. Thank you for completing this questionnaire, which should be returned by 28.2.91 to: Wendy Greenshields, 119 Belgrave, Southill, Weymouth, Dorset, DT4 9SN

THE NATIONAL CHILDBIRTH TRUST

The Research and Information Group of the NCT is conducting a survey into perineal trauma, and is distributing a questionnaire to mothers. We would also like the views and experiences of midwives, and would be grateful if practising midwives who regularly conduct deliveries would complete the following questionnaire. Please feel free to add any comments, which may be published anonymously in the report of this survey.

Please answer each question by putting the relevant number in each box, or 99 when question is not applicable.

1. What position do you hold? (1) Midwifery manager (2) Tutor ☐
    (3) Sister (4) Staff Midwife (5) Student Midwife
2. How long have you been working in your present position? ☐
    (1) More than 10 years (2) More than five years
    (3) Less than five years (4) Less than one year.
3. Which area do you work in? (1) Independent midwife (2) Community ☐
    (3) Consultant unit (4) Community and hospital as part of domino system.
4. In which county do you work?...
5. Approximately how many deliveries do you conduct each year? ☐
6. How independently do you feel able to practise? ☐
    (1) Very independently, I routinely make all my own decisions without consultation with anyone except the mother. (2) Fairly independently, I feel obliged to consult my superiors in the event of problems arising during labour. (3) Not very independently, I am obliged to follow unit policy.
7. How contented do you feel with the way you work? (1) Very contented ☐
    (2) Fairly contented (3) Not very contented.
8. If you answered (1) or (2) to the last question, what changes would make you more content?...
9. Do you feel able to allow mothers to adopt the positions that they feel ☐
    most comfortable with in *normal* labours?: (1) All the time (2) Some of the labour only (3) I follow my unit policy, which is...
10. Do you feel able to allow the mothers in your care to deliver in the positions they feel most comfortable with in *normal* labours? (1) With all mothers (2) With some mothers only (please say which)...
    (3) I am obliged to follow unit policy, which is
    ....
11. Do you have a favourite position for delivery that you encourage mothers ☐ to adopt (1) Yes (2) No. If Yes, please describe it and say why your prefer it...

12. How long do you allow a woman to push in the second stage of labour?
Primips (1) Up to one hour (2) More than one hour if condition of mother and baby allow (3) I am obliged to follow unit policy, which is ☐

....

Multips (1) Not more than 30-45 minutes. (2) Longer if condition of mother and baby allow. (3) I am obliged to follow unit policy, which is ☐

....

13. In the second stage of *normal* labour, are the women in your care ☐ mostly monitored by (1) Pinard stethoscope (2) Intermittent CTG using belts (3) Continuous CTG using belts (4) Continuous CTG using foetal scalp electrodes (5) Sonicaid.

14. In the second stage of labour, do you massage the perineum in order to ☐ 'iron' or to stretch it? (1) Yes (2) No

15. Do you use any oils or creams on the perineum during labour? ☐ (1) Yes (2) No. If yes, please state which and the benefit you think they have.

....

16. Do you think that mothers find perineal massage during labour: ☐ (1) Comforting, (2) Uncomfortable (3) Painful

17. Do you teach mothers to massage their own perineum during ☐ pregnancy? (1) Yes (2) No

18. If you do teach perineal massage to mothers, do you think they feel: ☐ (1) It is worth doing (2) It is not worth doing (3) It is unacceptable.

19. Do you think that perineal massage during pregnancy helps to ☐ preserve an intact perineum? (1) Yes (2) No (3) Don't know.

20. Do you think that perineal massage during labour helps to preserve ☐ an intact perineum? (1) Yes (2) No (3) Don't know

21. During the second stage of labour of a *normal* delivery, do you ☐ (1) Guard the perineum (2) Adopt a "hands off the perineum" policy (3) Use a different technique (please describe)

....

22. Do you encourage flexion of the foetal head, using your finger? ☐ (1) Yes (2) No

23. During the second stage of a *normal* labour, do you: (1) Encourage the ☐ mother to push with every contraction for as long as she can (2) Encourage her to push only when she wants to and only for as long as she wants (3) Not actively encourage her to do anything.

24. In a *normal* labour, do you perform episiotomy: (1) Routinely ☐ (2) Routinely for primigravid mothers (3) Only if necessary (4) Not at all if possible, preferring a tear to an episiotomy.

25. When episiotomy becomes necessary in *normal* deliveries, ☐ what do you consider to be the *most* common indication? (1) Rigid perineum

(2) Foetal distress (3) Maternal distress (4) Other (please state)
....

26. In the deliveries you have conducted in the last month, please state how many mothers had: (1) Episiotomies.......... (2) Unstitched tears ....(3) Stitched tears.......... (4) Episiotomies and tears.......... (5) Intact Perinea.......... (6) Tears of labia, urethra or clitoris..........

27. Do *you* routinely suture episiotomies? (1) Yes (2) No ☐

28. Do *you* routinely suture tears that require suturing? (1) Yes (2) No. ☐

29. If the answer to the above two questions is NO, is this because: ☐
(1) You have not yet received post-basic training in suturing (2) You are not yet competent to suture unsupervised. (3) Unit policy does not allow midwives to suture (4) You are allowed and are competent, but it is more usual for the doctor to do it.

30. If you do suture, which method do you use to close the skin? ☐
(1) Subcuticular suture (2) Interrupted sutures. (Please state why)
....

31. Which suturing material do you usually use to close the skin?
....
Please state why...

32. If a mother has an epidural that is still providing anaesthesia, do ☐
you before suturing: (1) Infiltrate perineum with normal saline (2) Infiltrate with local anaesthetic (3) Not infiltrate with anything?

33. Please state what measures you commonly use to relieve perineal discomfort and oedema. ....

34. Do you find it difficult to find time to treat perineal pain? ☐
(1) Yes, always (2) Sometimes (3) Never

35. Would you regard perineal pain as a (1) Major problem for mothers ☐
(2) Bit of a nuisance (3) Very minor problem?

36. If a perineum is infected, please state what measures you would commonly use to treat it.
....

37. Are you ever required to use substances which you regard as outdated ☐
or harmful? (1) Yes (2) No. If YES, please state which.
....

38. Do you, either before or after the birth, teach perineal hygiene to mothers (e.g. use of bidets, handling of sanitary towels etc)? (1) Yes (2) No

Thank you for completing this questionnaire. We would be most interested in any comments or suggestions that you would care to make regarding the care of the perineum during pregnancy, labour and postnatally. Please return by end of March to: Wendy Greenshields, 119 Belgrave, Southill, Weymouth, Dorset, DT4 9SN.